Contents

The Illustrated MRCP PACES Primer

Sebastian Zeki

This book is due for return on or before the last date shown below.

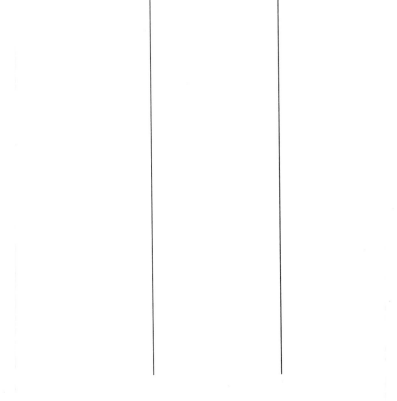

Radcliffe Publishing Ltd
18 Marcham Road
Abingdon
Oxon OX14 1AA
United Kingdom

www.radcliffe-oxford.com
Electronic catalogue and worldwide online ordering facility.

British Library Cataloguing in Publication Data

A catalogue record for this book is available from the British Library.

ISBN-13: 978 184619 349 1

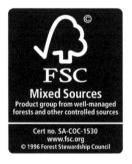

Typeset by Pindar NZ, Auckland, New Zealand
Printed and bound by Hobbs the Printers, Southampton, Hampshire, UK

Preface

The MRCP PACES examination remains a rigorous assessment of a doctor's ability to diagnose and treat a variety of common and uncommon conditions. Candidates will have seen many of the conditions before but equally so, many will be unfamiliar. The examination requires an easy familiarity with all the conditions and as such the candidate is supposed to have quick access to the knowledge required for any case in PACES.

This book is an attempt to ease the burden of reading for the candidate so he or she can concentrate on actually making diagnoses and examining patients in preparation. The emphasis is on one page layouts for each of the conditions with an abundance of memory techniques to help the candidate remember as much detail as possible. These include visual as well as verbal mnemonics. Emphasis is taken away from basic sciences as they are not tested in this examination. The book is, in essence, what you actually need to know in as easy a layout as possible.

We'd be grateful to hear readers' comments, ideas for layout/pictures and especially mnemonics that can be added in future editions. All published mnemonics will receive an acknowledgement. Please send your comments to editorial@radcliffemed.com

Sebastian Zeki
April 2009

About the Author

Sebastian Zeki is a gastroenterology registrar in London. He was born in London, went to Westminster School and then attended medical school at Gonville and Caius College, Cambridge and University College London. He qualified in 2001, has gained further degrees in medical informatics and computing whilst a doctor, and gained membership to the Royal College of Physicians in 2005. He is still working on his artwork ...

Acknowledgements

Many thanks to the following who checked and criticised:

Claire Sproson
Tom Shepherd
Damion Balmforth
Sophie Stevens.

Dedication

This book is dedicated to my mother and father and to Radha who spent a great deal of time laughing at the pictures ...

Abdominal System

Abdominal Masses
Ascites
Cirrhosis
Crohn's Disease
Haemochromatosis
Hepatomegaly
Primary Biliary Cirrhosis
Splenomegaly
Transplanted Kidney
Unilateral Palpable Kidney
Wilson's Disease

Abdominal Masses

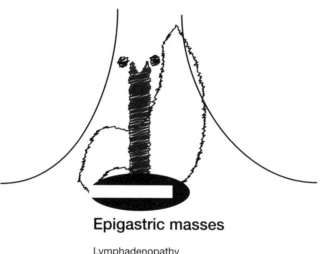

Epigastric masses

Lymphadenopathy
Masses arising from stomach
Pancreatic masses
AAA

Right iliac fossa mass

L ymph nodes
O vary (tumour)
C rohn's
C aecal cancer
C arcinoid
K idneys(transplanted or ectopic)
Amoebiasis

Actinomycosis
Abscesses (ileocaecal/ appendiceal)

Left iliac fossa mass

L ymph nodes
O varian cancer
C olonic – cancer
    Diverticular abscess, faeces
K idney (transplanted)

Ascites

Causes

Cirrhosis

CCF

Cancer (primary/ secondary)

Nephrotic

Constrictive pericarditis

TB

Budd–Chiari

NB: Separate into whether due to portal hypertension or not on the basis of the serum to ascites albumin gradient (SAAG) if >11 mmHg then due to PHTN the causes of which include cirrhosis/ Budd–Chiari, etc.

Features

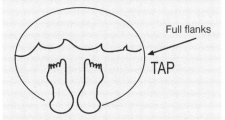

Full flanks

TAP

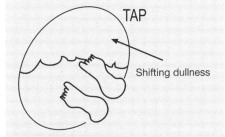

TAP

Shifting dullness

Complications

Respiratory problems
Spontaneous bacterial peritonitis

Management of ascites

Diuretic responsive ascites

(NaFD)
Na: Sodium restriction (<88 mmol/day)
F: Fluid restriction (if Na <120)
D: Diuretics (spironolactone + frusemide)

Diuretic resistant ascites

Paracentesis + albumin
Peritoneovenous shunt (LeVeen shunt)
TIPPS
Extracorporeal ultrafiltration
Liver transplantation

Cirrhosis

= Fibrosis with abnormal regenerating nodules

Causes

Autoimmune (PBC/CAH)

a**L**pha1 antitrypsin

I atrogenic (methyldopa/ methotrexate/
   amiodarone/ azathioprine)
Viral (Hep B)

Excess alcohol

R(haemoch**R**omatosis/ Wilson's)

Investigations that everyone should get

Bloods: FBC/ LFT/ PT Hep B/ Auto-Ab aFP/
   Ferritin
Fluids: Ascites
Radiology: Liver USS

Head

Jaundice
Encephalopathy
>5 spider naevi
   chest

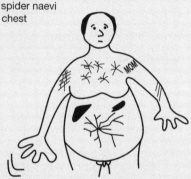

Hand signs

Clubbing
Dupuytren's
   contracture
Flap
Tattoos
Excoriation marks

Abdomen

Hepatosplenomegaly
   (not always)
Caput medusae
Testicular atrophy
Ascites
Bruising

Complications

G lucose low
R enal failure
E ncephalopathy
A scites
T hypo**T**ension

C oagulopathy
N utrition
G hypo**G**lycaemia
S epsis

TIPS

Once you have found chronic liver disease signs, you
know this patient has cirrhosis – now find a cause –
unkempt? (=EtOH), tattoos (=Hep B), massive
hepatomegaly (+PBC). If there are no chronic liver
disease signs, consider pre- (most likely in the exam) or
post-hepatic causes of jaundice.
   Pre-hepatic causes can be separated into congenital
(haemoglobin defects, e.g. sickle cell, or membrane
defects, etc.) or acquired.

Crohn's Disease

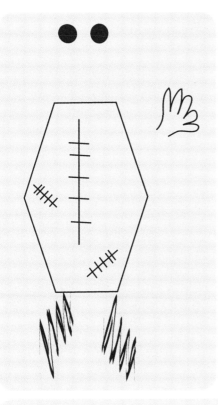

Features

Iritis

Clubbing

Multiple abdominal scars

Patient may be small (given steroids as a child)

Erythema nodosum

Pyoderma gangrenosum

Associations

Hepatobiliary: gallstones, steatosis
Eye: iritis, episcleritis
Signs of nutritional deficiencies, e.g. angular cheilosis (B12), anaemia, dermatitis (zinc)
Renal: oxalate stones

Investigations

Endoscopy
CT for abdominal masses
Barium follow through

Treatment

Metronidazole and ciprofloxacin
Elemental diet (controversial)
Steroids
Steroid-sparing agents (azathioprine/ methotrexate)
TNF-alpha antagonists

Haemochromatosis

Clinical manifestations

Liver disease (worse with Hep C and EtOH)
Hepatocellular carcinoma (increased x200)
Diabetes mellitus (selective for beta cell)
Arthropathy – (squared-off bone ends and
    hook-like osteophytes in the
    metacarpophalangeal (MCP) joints,
    particularly of the second and third
    MCP joints)
Heart disease (15% of HH)
Hypogonadism (usually pituitary origin)
Hypothyroidism (deposition in thyroid)
Extrahepatic cancer (controversial)
Susceptibility to specific infections
    (Listeria/ Yersinia (siderophage)/ *Vibrio
    vulnificus* (from uncooked seafood))
Manifestations in heterozygotes (rarely due
    to HH alone)

Secondary iron overload

Ineffective erythropoiesis (thalassaemia,
    aplastic anaemia, red cell aplasia, SCD)
Chronic liver disease
Excessive medicinal iron
Parenteral iron overload
Porphyria cutanea tarda

Investigations

Radiology
CT/MRI – liver is white/black respectively

Liver biopsy
To determine hepatic iron content

Familial things
Test all first degree relatives by PCR or
    HLA typing (A3)
• **Homozygote relative**
    12-monthly transferrin sats – venesect
    if more than 45%
• **Heterozygote relatives**
    Liver biopsies if LFTs abnormal.

Treatment

Bleed 1–2×/ week
Hct shouldn't fall >20% of previous
    level
Aim for ferritin between 25-50 nh/mL
Avoid Vit C/ uncooked seafood

Results

Improves everything except
• advanced cirrhosis
• arthropathy
• hypogonadism

Prognosis

Cardiac failure = bad sign
Survival normal if no diabetes/liver
    damage
If cirrhotic 70% 5-year survival
One-third of cirrhosis die from HCC

Hepatomegaly

Causes

CCF
Cirrhosis ⎤ 3 Cs
Cancer (1°/2°) ⎦

Infiltration

Reticuloendothelial
(e.g. leukaemia)

Hepatoma (H)
Infections (EBV/Hep B) (I)
Budd–Chiari (B)

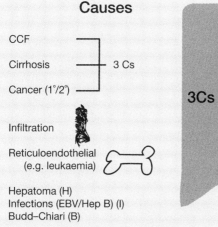

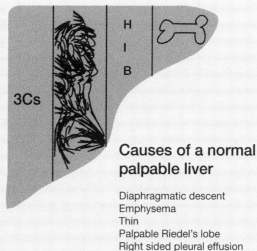

H
I
B

3Cs

Causes of a normal palpable liver

Diaphragmatic descent
Emphysema
Thin
Palpable Riedel's lobe
Right sided pleural effusion

Characteristics

Pulsatile liver
Bruits
Venous hum
Friction rub

Tricuspid regurgitation
EtOH or 1°/ 2° cancer
Portal hypertension
Fitz–Hugh–Curtis syndrome

Tips

Hepatomegaly is most likely to be due to the 3Cs in the exam. Therefore

• look for the JVP for CCF
• look for lymphadenopathy/ cachexia/ rough liver edge in cancer
• look for signs of chronic liver disease in cirrhosis

Primary Biliary Cirrhosis

Associations

Glomerulonephritis   Renal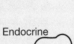

Hypertrophic
   osteoarthropathy
Arthralgia
Sclerodactyly   Rheum
Raynaud's
SLE

TP   Derm
Vitiligo

Thyroid disease   Endocrine
Addison's

Features

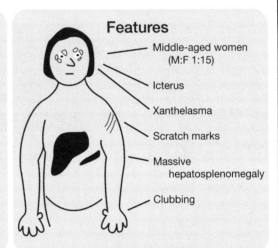

- Middle-aged women (M:F 1:15)
- Icterus
- Xanthelasma
- Scratch marks
- Massive hepatosplenomegaly
- Clubbing

Phase

1. Increased AMA only
2. Increased AMA and LFTs
3. Increased AMA, LFTs and pruritis
4. Decompensated PBC

Prognosis

>12 yrs

8–12 yrs
5–10 yrs
3–5 yrs

Histopathology

1. Biliary duct epithelial damage with lymphocyte infiltration +/– granulomas (fluid lesions)
2. Piecemeal necrosis
3. Bridging fibrosis
4. Cirrhosis

Investigations

Cholestatic LFTs
Clotting (until late stages)
Cholesterol increased
AMA E2 – specific to PBC so often no need for liver biopsy

Complications

Vit ADEK deficiency
Metabolic bone disease (osteoporosis plus malacia)
Hypercholesterolaemia and xanthomas
Malabsorption (due to decreased bile salt secretion)
Hypothyroidism (in 20%)
Anaemia

Treatment

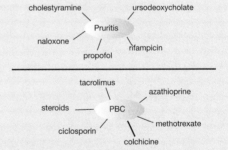

ADEK – stops bone problems (as per osteoporosis)
Lipid lowering – no need
UDCA – 30% RR decrease to ALF
Liver transplantation = 50% 5-year survival
Monitoring = 6/12 alpha fetoprotein + USS
Can recur
Azathioprine/steroids – marginal improvement

Splenomegaly

Massive

All the Ms

Myeloproliferative
Malaria
Myelofibrosis

+ Gaucher's
+ Kala-azar

Moderate

Cirrhosis
Lymphoproliferative

Mild

I   Inflammatory
(Sarcoid/ SLE/ Rheumatoid arthritis)

Infection
(hepatitis/ EBV/ bacterial
   endocarditis)

Haematological
(ITP/ spherocytosis/ PAU)

Causes of asplenia

Congenital
Acquired
After splenectomy
Sickle cell disease
Hereditary spherocytosis

Asplenia precautions

At risk of:
Neisseria meningitidis
Strep. pneumoniae
Haemophilus influenzae B
Babesiasis
Malaria

Vaccination required

Pneumococcal vaccine
HiB
Meningococcal A and C

Reasons for splenectomy

Haematological disorders

Idiopathic
   thrombocytopenic
   purpura (ITP)
Hereditary spherocytosis
Idiopathic autoimmune
   haemolytic anaemia
Felty's syndrome
Thalassaemia
Sarcoidosis
Sickle cell disease
Gaucher's disease
Congenital and acquired
   hemolytic anaemia
Thrombotic
   thrombocytopenic
   purpura

Malignancies

Hodgkin's/
   Non-Hodgkin's
   lymphoma
Hairy cell leukaemia
Lymphoproliferative
   disorders

Miscellaneous

Splenic artery aneurysm
Splenic cysts/ abscesses
Trauma

Transplanted Kidney

Causes of chronic renal failure (and therefore need for transplantation)

G lomerulonephritis
P yelonephritis
C ystic disease
H ypertension
D iabetes mellitus
A myloidosis
M yeloma

Examination

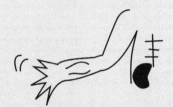

Tacrolimus tremor
AV fistula (?bruit/ ?recently punctured?)
Laparotomy scar
Iliac fossa mass

Matching considerations

HLA DR>B>A
ABO

Complications of renal transplant

Coronary artery disease
Opportunistic infections
Hypertension
Lymphoma and skin cancer
Glomerulonephritis
Steroid complications

Contraindications

For donors

Pre-existing renal disease
Disease of unknown aetiology   **?**
Ischaemic heart disease
Hypertension with end-organ damage

For recipients

No infections (I)

Normal uro-genital system (UG)
Significant GI disease controlled (GI)
Autoimmune disease quiescent (I)

Post transplant medications

Steroids
Tacrolimus
MMF
Azathioprine
Ciclosporin

Causes of rejection

Opportunistic infection
Premature CAD
Hypertension
Lymphomas and skin cancer
Glomerulonephritis
Steroid complications

Unilateral Palpable Kidney

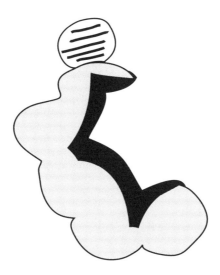

Causes

Adult polycystic kidney disease/ renal cyst

Renal cell cancer

Hydronephrosis (wide pelvis on picture)

Hypertrophied solitary functioning kidney

Wilson's Disease

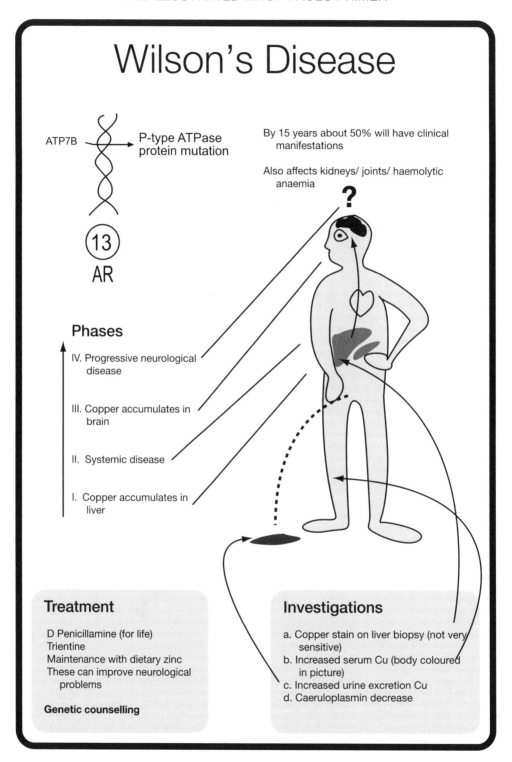

ATP7B → P-type ATPase protein mutation

(13)

AR

By 15 years about 50% will have clinical manifestations

Also affects kidneys/ joints/ haemolytic anaemia

?

Phases

IV. Progressive neurological disease

III. Copper accumulates in brain

II. Systemic disease

I. Copper accumulates in liver

Treatment

D Penicillamine (for life)
Trientine
Maintenance with dietary zinc
These can improve neurological problems

Genetic counselling

Investigations

a. Copper stain on liver biopsy (not very sensitive)
b. Increased serum Cu (body coloured in picture)
c. Increased urine excretion Cu
d. Caeruloplasmin decrease

Cardiovascular System

Aortic Regurgitation

High pitched/ left sternal edge/ early diastole. Also at base if severe
Severity signs include
1. Soft S2
2. S3
3. Wide pulse pressure
4. Lengthened murmur
5. Austin Flint murmur (as on murmur diagram)

Causes of chronic AR

Marfan's
Ankylosing spondylitis
Rheumatic fever
Rheumatoid arthritis
Infective endocarditis
Syphilis

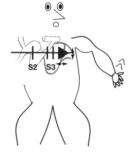

Features

Apex displaced downwards
3rd heart sound
Soft diastolic high pitched
   murmur at the left sternal
   edge
Mid diastolic murmur at apex
Signs of pulmonary
   hypertension

Associated signs

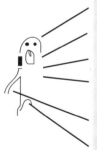

de Musset's sign – head nodding

Müller's sign – dancing uvula

Corrigan's sign – Corrigan's carotids

Austin–Flint murmur – apical/ low pitched/ diastolic. Due to
   anterior mitral cusp vibration in regurgitant jet

Quincke's sign – pulsating nail beds

Traube's sign ('femoral pistol shots' – remember Traube = trouble)

Hill's sign – higher systolic in leg than arm – in moderate AR
   difference is 20 mmHg/ mild 20–40/ severe >60

Surgical indications

EF <0.5 and >0.25 and symptomatic
No more than 55 mm dimension –
Reduction in exercise ejection fraction
   of >5%

Treatment

Nil if normal blood pressure/
   mild AR/ normal LV
Nifedipine (delays need for
   surgery and better result if
   need surgery later)
Surgery as above

Aortic Stenosis

Presentation

Dyspnoea
Syncope (due to LV unable to contract vs closed
    valve/ post-exercise peripheral dilatation with
    no rise in CO)
Arrhythmias
Angina
Sudden death

Aortic stenosis vs sclerosis
  – in latter no radiation
Normovolaemic pulse
Apex undisplaced

Causes

<60 yrs – congenital/ RF
60–75 calcified bicuspid valve
>75 yrs degenerative
    calcification

Pulsus parvus et tardus
  – reduced volume/
  delayed upstroke

Markers of severity

Soft S2
Displaced apex
Delayed peak of murmur
CHF
S4
Reversed split S2
Narrow pulse pressure

S1
ejection
click

S2

soft
narrow
or
reverse
split

S4

APEX

Complications

LVF
Infective endocarditis

ECG – ST changes/ LVH
ECHO – LVH/ calcified valves/ valve
    gradient

CXR – valve calcification/ post
    stenotic dilatation of aorta
Catheterisation – mitral and aortic
    valves and coronary arteries

Valve Area

(Mild = >1.5 cm^2
Moderate = 1–1.5 cm^2
Severe = <1 cm^2)

Surgical indications

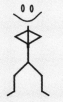

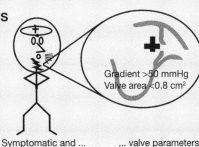

Gradient >50 mmHg
Valve area <0.8 cm^2

Asymptomatic – no surgery   Symptomatic and ...   ... valve parameters

Coarctation of the Aorta

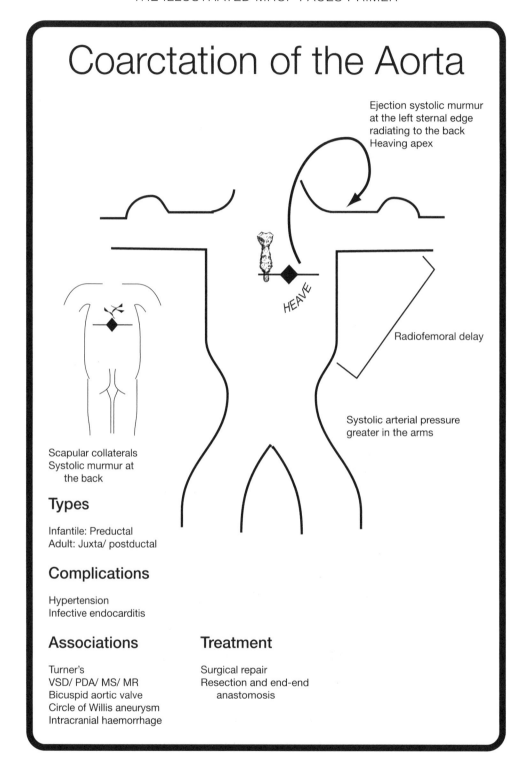

Ejection systolic murmur at the left sternal edge radiating to the back
Heaving apex

HEAVE

Radiofemoral delay

Systolic arterial pressure greater in the arms

Scapular collaterals
Systolic murmur at the back

Types

Infantile: Preductal
Adult: Juxta/ postductal

Complications

Hypertension
Infective endocarditis

Associations

Turner's
VSD/ PDA/ MS/ MR
Bicuspid aortic valve
Circle of Willis aneurysm
Intracranial haemorrhage

Treatment

Surgical repair
Resection and end-end
    anastomosis

Congestive Cardiac Failure

Features

Raised JVP
Enlarged liver/ swollen ankles (right heart
    failure signs)
S3/ S4
Displaced apex
RV heave
MR and/or TR

Causes of heart failure

H TN
E ndocrine
A naemia
R heumatic heart disease
T oxins

F ailure to take medications
A rrhythmias
I nfection/ ischaemia
L ung problems
E lectrolytes
D iet

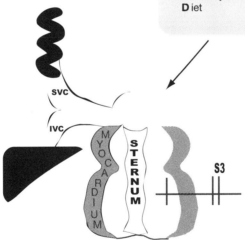

Treatment

Diuretics
ACEI
Digoxin
Nitrates
Beta-blockers

Trial

RALES
CONSENSUS/ SOLVD/ VeHeFT-II
PROVED/ RADIANCE

For dilated cardiomyopathy (MERIT/ CIBIS-11/ BEST)

Constrictive Pericarditis

Causes

C onnective tissue disorders
O
N
S
T uberculosis
R adiation therapy
I
C ancer
T
I
V
E

Features

Prominent x and y descent of JVP
which rises with inspiration
Can't palpate apex
Diastolic pericardial knock
Signs of right heart failure

Treatment

Surgery – resection of pericardium

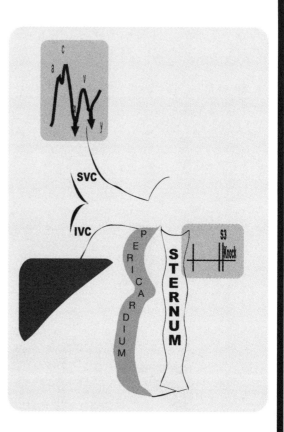

Pericardial Rub

Causes

TB
Coxsackie A/B
Chronic renal failure
MI
Trauma

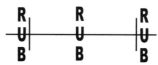

Treatment

NSAIDs
Steroids
Treat underlying condition
Colchicine

Dextrocardia

Dextrocardia

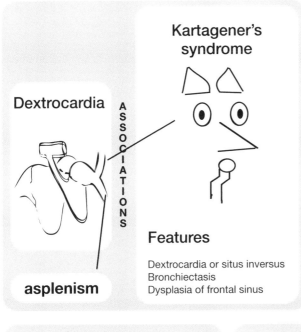

asplenism

Kartagener's syndrome

Features

Dextrocardia or situs inversus
Bronchiectasis
Dysplasia of frontal sinus

ASSOCIATIONS

Dextroversion

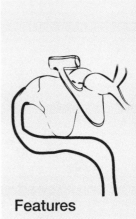

Features

Right sided apex
Left stomach
Left descending aorta

Situs Inversus

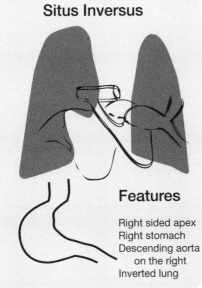

Features

Right sided apex
Right stomach
Descending aorta
   on the right
Inverted lung

Levoversion

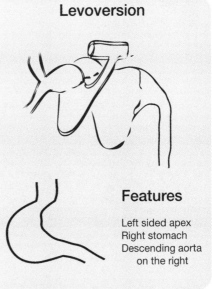

Features

Left sided apex
Right stomach
Descending aorta
   on the right

Ebstein's Anomaly

Tricuspid valve is low in the R ventricle
atrialisation

Cyanosis occurs via R-L shunt at atrial level – via
ASD/ patent foramen ovale

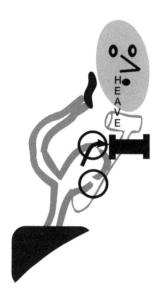

Clinical findings

Cyanosis
Raised JVP
L parasternal heave
Pansystolic murmur loudest in expiration
Hepatomegaly

Investigations

ECG – RBBB/ long PR/ P pulmonale
CXR – large RA with oligaemia
ECHO – abnorm tricuspid
No place for catheterisation

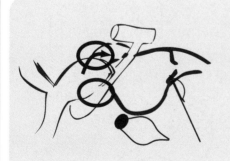

Treatment

Surgical therapy

1. Valve replacement with ASD repair

2. Annuloplasty with plication of atrialised
   part of R ventricle

Eisenmenger's Syndrome

= Pulmonary hypertension with right to left shunt

Features

Clubbing and cyanosis
a-waves in the JVP
v-waves if TR
Pansystolic TR murmur
Pulmonary regurgitation
Underlying murmur that causes Eisenmenger's

a-waves

Complications

Haemoptysis
RV failure
CVA
Brain abscess
Bleeding and thrombosis
Infective endocarditis

v-waves if TR

P2

VSD – Single second sound
ASD – Fixed wide second sound
PDA – Reversed split of second sound

SVC

IVC

Aorta

M
Y
O
C
A
R
D
I
U
M

ASD

VSD

PDA

Poor prognostics

Right heart failure
Syncope
Any evidence of decreased
    cardiac output

Treatment

Phlebotomy for polycythaemia
IV epoprostenol
Heart–lung transplantation

Fallot's Tetralogy

Anatomy

Pulmonary stenosis
VSD with R-L shunt
RVH
Dextroverted aorta overriding the VSD

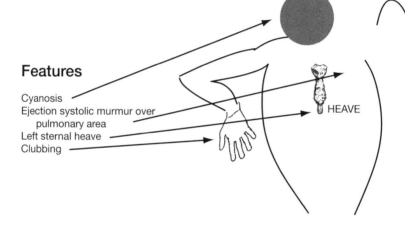

Features

Cyanosis
Ejection systolic murmur over
    pulmonary area
Left sternal heave
Clubbing

HEAVE

Treatment

Total correction <1 yr of age and second
    stage operation >2 years
Blalock–Taussig = graft between left
    subclavian and left pulmonary artery

Complications

Cyanosis and syncope
Cerebral abscess
Endocarditis
Paradoxical emboli
Strokes

Hypertension

Investigations

FBC/ U&Es
Fasting lipids
Uric acid

ECG/ CXR

Urine for sugar/
    albumin and
    specific gravity

Other tests

Renal digital
    subtraction
    angiography
24 hr urinary
    catecholamines
Overnight dex
    suppression test

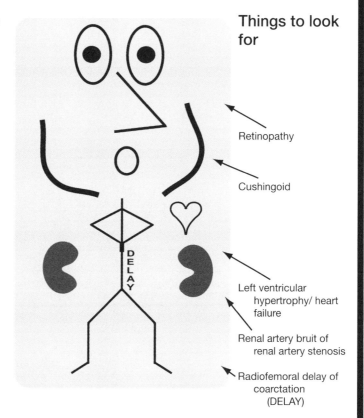

Things to look for

Retinopathy

Cushingoid

Left ventricular
    hypertrophy/ heart
    failure

Renal artery bruit of
    renal artery stenosis

Radiofemoral delay of
    coarctation
    (DELAY)

Causes of blood pressure difference between the arms and the legs

Coarctation
PDA
Dissection
Arterial occlusion
Thoracic outlet syndrome

Hypertrophic Obstructive Cardiomyopathy

It just can't relax – diastolic dysfunction

Implicated genes

1. Beta myosin heavy chain gene
2. Alpha tropomyosin
3. Cardiac troponin T

Features

Bifid carotid
a-wave in JVP
Pansystolic murmur at the apex
Ejection systolic murmur at left
    sternal edge
Louder on standing, softer on
    squatting

Associations

Friedreich's ataxia

Presents with

Dizziness
SOB
Sudden death

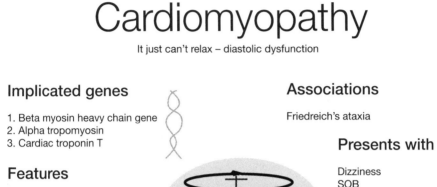
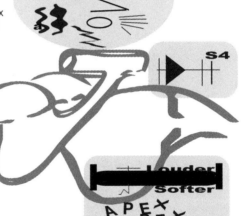

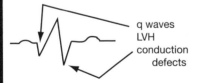

q waves
LVH
conduction
    defects

ECHO findings   Mr Sam Ash

Mitral regurgitation using Doppler – MR
Systolic – anterior motion of the mitral valve – SAM
Asymmetric septa/ hypertrophy – ASH

Treatment

Drugs – VBad – Verapamil/ Beta-blocker/ Amiodarone/ Diuretic
Pacing – DDD/ dual chamber
Surgery – myomectomy/ myotomy – symptomatic treament only
Counselling

Infective Endocarditis

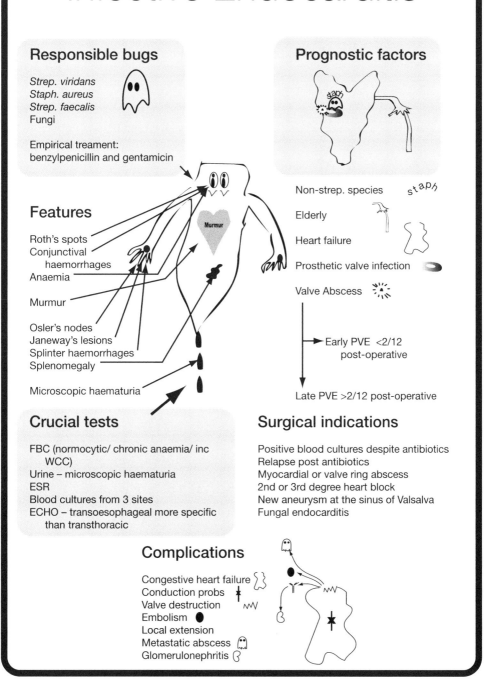

Responsible bugs

Strep. viridans
Staph. aureus
Strep. faecalis
Fungi

Empirical treament:
benzylpenicillin and gentamicin

Prognostic factors

Non-strep. species
Elderly
Heart failure
Prosthetic valve infection
Valve Abscess

→ Early PVE <2/12
         post-operative

Late PVE >2/12 post-operative

Features

Roth's spots
Conjunctival
     haemorrhages
Anaemia

Murmur

Osler's nodes
Janeway's lesions
Splinter haemorrhages
Splenomegaly

Microscopic haematuria

Crucial tests

FBC (normocytic/ chronic anaemia/ inc
     WCC)
Urine – microscopic haematuria
ESR
Blood cultures from 3 sites
ECHO – transoesophageal more specific
     than transthoracic

Surgical indications

Positive blood cultures despite antibiotics
Relapse post antibiotics
Myocardial or valve ring abscess
2nd or 3rd degree heart block
New aneurysm at the sinus of Valsalva
Fungal endocarditis

Complications

Congestive heart failure
Conduction probs
Valve destruction
Embolism
Local extension
Metastatic abscess
Glomerulonephritis

JVP

Distinguish arterial pulse from venous pulse by:

1. Pulse is better felt than seen
2. Hepato–jugular reflux
3. JVP fills on inspiration
4. JVP has an upper level

Another way of remembering the causes ...

P ericardial effusion
Q uantity of fluid raised (i.e. fluid overload)
R ight heart failure
S VC obstruction
T ricuspid regurg/ stenosis/ tamponade

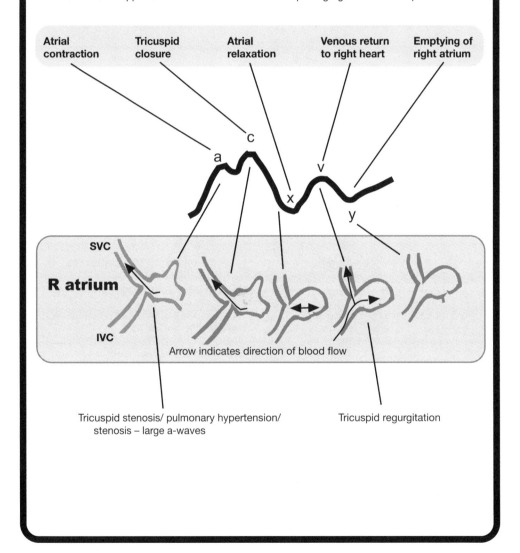

Atrial contraction | **Tricuspid closure** | **Atrial relaxation** | **Venous return to right heart** | **Emptying of right atrium**

SVC

R atrium

IVC

Arrow indicates direction of blood flow

Tricuspid stenosis/ pulmonary hypertension/ stenosis – large a-waves

Tricuspid regurgitation

Mitral Regurgitation

Causes of chronic MR

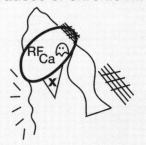

Mitral valve prolapse
Rheumatic heart disease **(RF)**
Left ventricular dilatation

Coronary artery disease
Annular calcification (Ca)
Infective endocarditis
Papillary muscle dysfunction **(X)**

Cardiomyopathy

Connective tissue disorders

Features

Peripheral pulse normal or jerky
Apex down and out
Soft S1
S3
Pansystolic murmur radiating to the axilla
and loudest on expiration
Pulmonary hypertension signs

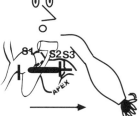

Severity correlates with
left ventricular size

Signs of clinical severity

Large ventricle
Signs of pulmonary
hypertension

Investigations

ECG (MI/LVH/AF)
CXR (LA and LV enlarged)
ECHO (note LA/LV/ejection
fraction)
Catheterisation (for aortic
valve disease/ coronary
artery disease)

Acute MR

Causes

1. Acute (MI) papillary muscle
rupture

2. Endocarditis

3. Trauma

4. Myxomatous degeneration

Associations

1. Ostium primum atrial septal defect
2. Partial atrioventricular canal
3. Corrected transposition of the great arteries

Surgical indications

1. Severe symptoms   2.

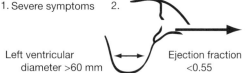

Left ventricular
diameter >60 mm

Ejection fraction
<0.55

Mitral Stenosis

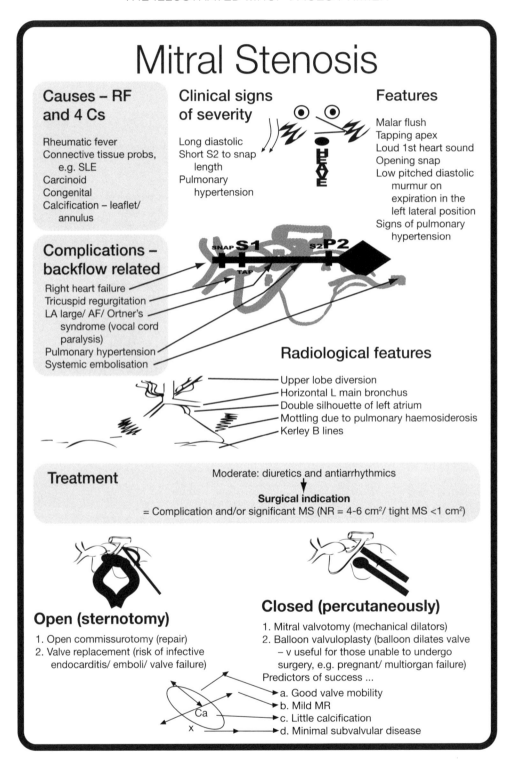

Causes – RF and 4 Cs

Rheumatic fever
Connective tissue probs,
    e.g. SLE
Carcinoid
Congenital
Calcification – leaflet/
    annulus

Complications – backflow related

Right heart failure
Tricuspid regurgitation
LA large/ AF/ Ortner's
    syndrome (vocal cord
    paralysis)
Pulmonary hypertension
Systemic embolisation

Clinical signs of severity

Long diastolic
Short S2 to snap
    length
Pulmonary
    hypertension

Features

Malar flush
Tapping apex
Loud 1st heart sound
Opening snap
Low pitched diastolic
    murmur on
    expiration in the
    left lateral position
Signs of pulmonary
    hypertension

SNAP S1   **S2 P2**
TAP

Radiological features

Upper lobe diversion
Horizontal L main bronchus
Double silhouette of left atrium
Mottling due to pulmonary haemosiderosis
Kerley B lines

Treatment

Moderate: diuretics and antiarrhythmics

Surgical indication
= Complication and/or significant MS (NR = 4-6 cm^2/ tight MS <1 cm^2)

Open (sternotomy)

1. Open commissurotomy (repair)
2. Valve replacement (risk of infective
    endocarditis/ emboli/ valve failure)

Closed (percutaneously)

1. Mitral valvotomy (mechanical dilators)
2. Balloon valvuloplasty (balloon dilates valve
    – v useful for those unable to undergo
    surgery, e.g. pregnant/ multiorgan failure)
Predictors of success ...
    a. Good valve mobility
    b. Mild MR
    c. Little calcification
    d. Minimal subvalvular disease

Ca

Mitral Valve Prolapse

aka Barlow's syndrome/ click-murmur syndrome/ floppy mitral valve

Associations

Marfan's
Rheumatic heart disease
Ischaemic heart disease
Cardiomyopathy
Ehlers–Danlos
SLE
Psoriatic arthritis
Ebstein's anomaly

Features

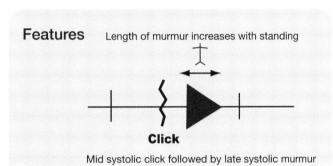

Length of murmur increases with standing

Click

Mid systolic click followed by late systolic murmur

Complications

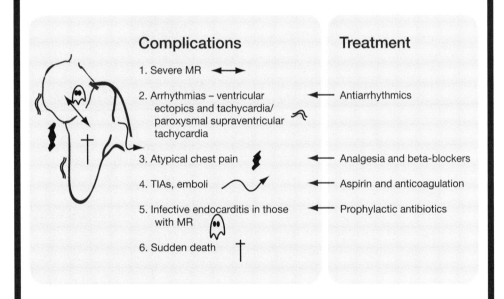

1. Severe MR

2. Arrhythmias – ventricular ectopics and tachycardia/ paroxysmal supraventricular tachycardia

3. Atypical chest pain

4. TIAs, emboli

5. Infective endocarditis in those with MR

6. Sudden death

Treatment

Antiarrhythmics

Analgesia and beta-blockers

Aspirin and anticoagulation

Prophylactic antibiotics

Mixed Aortic Valve Lesion

Causes

1. Rheumatic heart disease
2. Bicuspid aortic valve

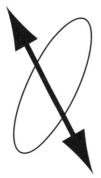

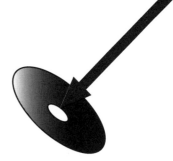

Aortic regurgitation

Collapsing pulse/ wide pulse pressure

Aortic stenosis

Small pulse volume/ narrow pulse pressure

Treatment

Dominant AR – Delay op until LV dysfunction on ECHO
Dominant AS – Operate even in mild disease

Mixed Mitral Valve Disease

(a question of finding the dominant lesion)

Cause – Rheumatic fever

MS vs **MR**

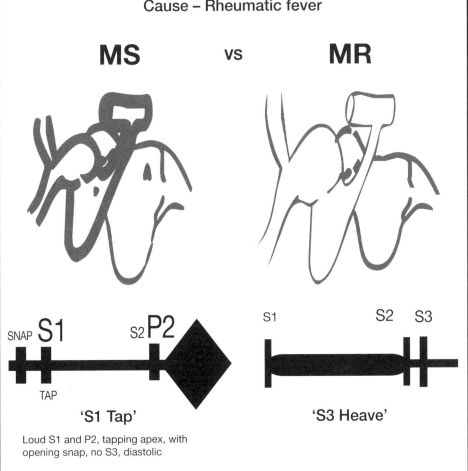

'S1 Tap'

Loud S1 and P2, tapping apex, with
opening snap, no S3, diastolic

'S3 Heave'

NB: MR + diastolic rumble + larger L atrium = no significant MS

Patent Ductus Arteriosus

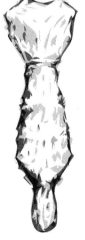

Second intercostal space

Features

Murmur in 2nd intercostal space
Machinery murmur through systole and
    diastole
Inaudible second heart sound

Complications

CCF
IE
Portal hypertension with reversal and cyanosis of the lower
    limbs
Ductus rupture

Associations

VSD
Pulmonary stenosis
Coarctation

Treatment

PGE
Rashkind PDA occluder
Surgery if large shunt present

Permanent Cardiac Pacemaker

For ...
Symptomatic bradycardia
Mobitz type 2
Complete heart block

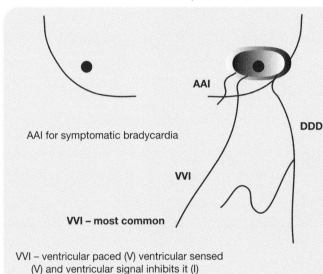

AAI

AAI for symptomatic bradycardia

DDD

VVI

VVI – most common

DDD – sick sinus syndrome
Won't pace if senses spontaneous signal in either atrium or ventricle. Wherever signal is missing it will pace – either atrium or ventricle

VVI – ventricular paced (V) ventricular sensed (V) and ventricular signal inhibits it (I)

Driving after one month of pacemaker working
Insurers and DVLA to be aware

Indications for implantable cardiac defibrillators

Cardiac arrest from VT

Spontaneous sustained VT

Syncope with inducible VT

Non-sustained VT with CAD

Complications

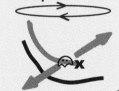

Erosion through skin

Infection

Lead displacement

Pacemaker malfunction **✗**

Pacemaker syndrome (low cardiac output causing dizziness due to loss of atrial kick)

Primary Pulmonary Hypertension

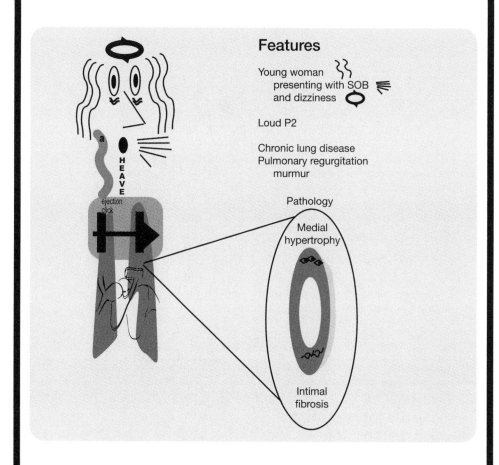

Features

Young woman
   presenting with SOB
   and dizziness

Loud P2

Chronic lung disease
Pulmonary regurgitation
   murmur

Pathology

Medial
hypertrophy

Intimal
fibrosis

a

HEAVE

ejection
click

Investigations

Pulmonary function
   tests
ECG
CXR
ECHO

Treatment

The pulmonary PACT

1. **P** rostaglandin
2. **A** nticoagulation
3. **C** alcium channel blockers
4. **T** ransplantation (heart 'n' lung)
5. Atrial septostomy

Prosthetic Valves

Mitral prosthetic valves

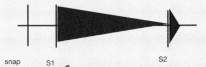

snap   S1   S2
metallic

Systolic murmur normal
Diastolic murmur normal

Always mechanical unless anticoagulation
contraindicated – is then bioprosthetic

Aortic prosthetic valves

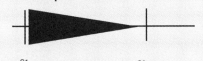

S1   S2
metallic

Systolic murmur normal
Diastolic murmur abnormal

Mechanical in the young – porcine in the
old when life expectancy <valve life
expectancy

Prosthetic valve complications

Valve dysfunction due to
a. Structural fracture/ poppet
   escape/ cuspal tear/
   calcification
b. Paravalvular leak/ suture
   or tissue entrapment
c. Haemolysis
d. Bleeding (anticoags)
e. Endocarditis
f. Thromboembolism

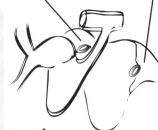

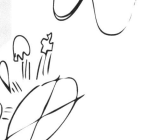

Valve types

1. Mechanical

Starr–Edwards – high
   haemolysis rates
Bjork–Shiley – single
   tilting disc
St. Jude – double tilting
   disc

2. Xenograft

Porcine (Carpentier–
   Edwards, Hancock,
   Wessex)
Pericardial valves
   (Ionescu–Shiley,
   Hancock)

3. Homografts

i.e. cadaveric aortic/
   pulmonary valves

Valve choices

a. Anticoagulants contraindicated/   bioprosthetic
   short life span
b. Over 70 needing aortic valve   bioprosthetic
   replacement
c. Pregnant   bioprosthetic (no warfarin – teratogen) vs mechanical
                                      (no degeneration) – still being debated
d. Atrial fibrillation   mechanical as needs warfarinisation anyway

Pulmonary Stenosis

Causes are congenital or carcinoid

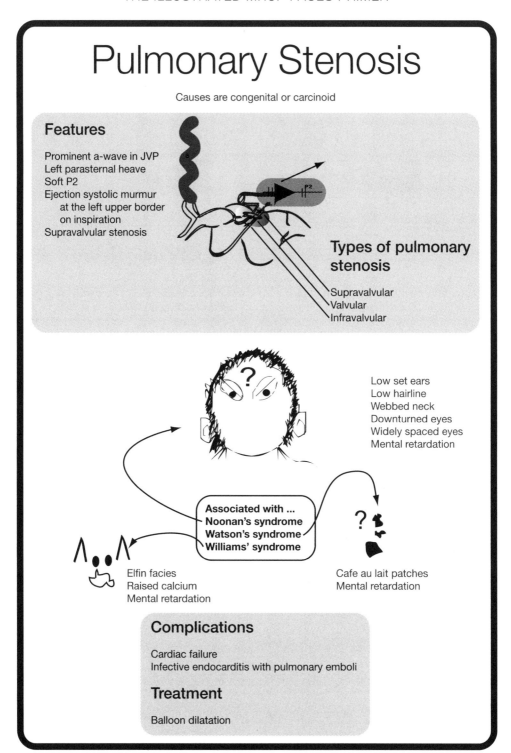

Features

Prominent a-wave in JVP
Left parasternal heave
Soft P2
Ejection systolic murmur
    at the left upper border
    on inspiration
Supravalvular stenosis

Types of pulmonary stenosis

Supravalvular
Valvular
Infravalvular

Low set ears
Low hairline
Webbed neck
Downturned eyes
Widely spaced eyes
Mental retardation

Associated with ...
Noonan's syndrome
Watson's syndrome
Williams' syndrome

Elfin facies
Raised calcium
Mental retardation

Cafe au lait patches
Mental retardation

Complications

Cardiac failure
Infective endocarditis with pulmonary emboli

Treatment

Balloon dilatation

Tricuspid Regurgitation

Features

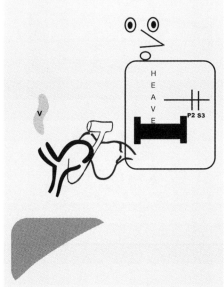

Causes

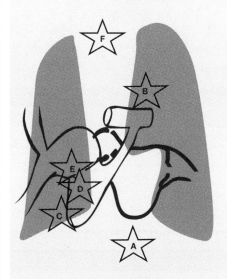

a. Congestive cardiac failure
b. Pulmonary hypertension
c. Endomyocardial fibrosis
d. Infarction of right ventricular papillary muscles
e. Valvular problems – Ebstein's anomaly/ rheumatic heart disease assoc with aortic/ mitral valve disease/ IVDU endocarditis/ tricuspid valve prolapse
f. Outside cardiopulmonary carcinoid/ blunt trauma to the heart

Peripheral cyanosis
v-waves
Left parasternal heave
Loud P2
Pansystolic murmur at left sternal edge

Treatment

Valve replacement
Valve plication or annuloplasty

Ventricular Septal Defect

Commonest congenital cardiac condition (usually in membranous part)
Also due to MIs (interventricular septal rupture)

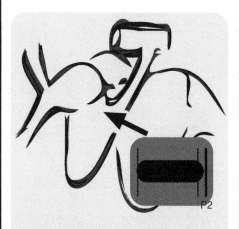

Types

1. Supracristal

2. Infracristal
   Maladie de Roger
   Swiss Cheese
   Gerbode defect

Features

Pansystolic at left sternal edge with
  palpable thrill
Occasional aortic regurg if defect is next
  to annulus
Can develop pulmonary hypertension

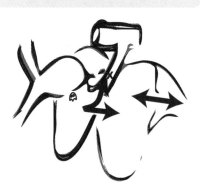

Complications

1. Congestive cardiac failure
2. R ventricular outflow tract obstruction
3. Aortic regurgitation
4. Infective endocarditis
5. Eisenmenger's

Syndromes of which VSD is a part

Fallot's
Truncus arteriosus
Double outlet right ventricle

Tests

Doppler ECHO
Cardiac catheterisation
  and angiography

Treatment

Surgery if LVF or
  pulmonary hypertension

Dermatology

Alopecia Areata

Associations

Autoimmune
Down's
Hypogammaglob

Treatment

Steroids
PUVA
Minoxidil
Dithranol

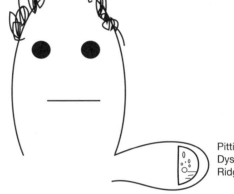

Pitting
Dystrophy
Ridging

Non-scarring, well defined hair loss patch.
Exclamation mark hairs at the advancing edge

Bullous Diseases

Causes

Porphyria cutanea tarda
Paraneoplastic
Other (friction/ insect bites/
    burns/ drugs/ impetigo/
    contact dermatitis)
Autoimmune ➡

Pemphigus (Nikolsky's sign – superficial pressing
    on blister causes easy separation). Two types
    – foliaceous and vulgaris (begins in the mouth)
Pemphigoid (tense blisters in flexural areas in
    old-IgG and C3 in lamina lucida)
IgA mediated
Bullous erythema multiforme
Epidermolysis bullosa acquisita
Dermatitis herpetiformis

Association

Gluten sensitivity
Thyroid
    dysfunction
Lymphoma

Investigations

Skin biopsy
D2 biopsy
Anti-endomysial
    antibodies

Anti-gliadin antibodies
Tissue transglutaminase
HLA-B8
HLA-DRw3

Treatment

As per coeliac
    disease
Dapsone for
    itching

Management of autoimmune blistering condition

1. Steroids (except IgA) – oral not topical
2. Other immunosuppressants (with steroids)
3. Dapsone (IgA/ dermatitis herpet – expect 48 hr response)
4. Gluten free diet (dermatitis herpetiformis)
5. Other therapies – colchicine for IgA/ extracorporeal absorption
    antibodies in pemphigus/ tetracycline in bullous pemphigoid
6. Plasmapheresis
7. Chrysotherapy (gold)

Varicella Zoster Syndrome (shingles)

Features

Dermatomal distribution
Appears as crops of blisters

Investigation

Tzanck smear (get
multinucleated giant cells)

Complications

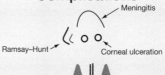

Meningitis
Ramsay–Hunt
Corneal ulceration
Pneumonia

Management

Topical idovudine if
    caught early
Pain relief
IV aciclovir if HIV
Interferon if cancer

Facial Problems 1

Seborrhoeic dermatitis

Risk factors

HIV
Parkinson's
Stroke

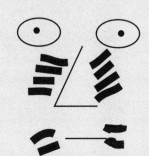

Features

Greasy skin around mouth
and nose overlying
    erythematous patches

Treatment

Topical glucocorticoids
Coal tar and salicylic acid
Selenium sulpiride shampoo
Oral ketoconazole

Acne vulgaris

Features

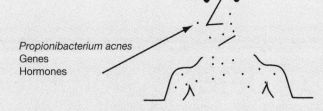

Propionibacterium acnes
Genes
Hormones

Blackheads
    (comedones) over
    face/upper
    chest/upper arms
Whiteheads
Cysts
Greasiness

Treatment

Wash once a day
Avoid Turkish baths and saunas

Sebum reduction: oestrogens, anti-androgens
Propionibacterium reduction: tetracycline/
    doxycycline/ isotretinoin
Inflammation reduction: topical or systemic
    steroids

Facial Problems 2

Sturge–Weber syndrome

Features

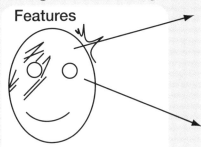

Port wine stain (1st and 2nd
    division of Vth cranial nerve
    with hypertrophy)
Neuro probs
Eye probs

Neuro probs

Jacksonian epilepsy
Contralat hemianopia
Hemisensory
    disturbance
Hemiparesis/ anopia
Low IQ

Treatment

Anti-epileptics
Ophthalmological
    review
Photothermolysis

Eye probs

Choroidal angioma
Glaucoma
Buphthalmos
Optic atrophy
Haemangioma of
    episclera and iris

Xanthelasma – in any condition with raised cholesterol

Causes

DM
Hypothyroid
Nephrotic
Cholestasis
XS EtOH
OCP

Treatment

Lifestyle advice
Dietary advice
Avoid EtOH/ smoking/ oestrogen/ thiazides
Control hypertension and diabetes
Exercise
Decrease lipids

Eruptive xanthomata
Seen in all except IIa

Palmar xanthomata
Type III

Tendon xanthomata
Homozygotes have these at birth – die by 30
    years old
Heterozygotes – 50% present at same age
In familial hyperchol (IIa, III) – (due to LDL
    receptor defect)

Lipoatrophy

Causes

Mesangiocapillary GN
    (type 2)
Localised scleroderma
Morphoea

Chronic relapsing
    panniculitis
NNRTIs and PIs
    (antiretrovirals)

Hereditary Haemorrhagic Telangiectasia

Genetics

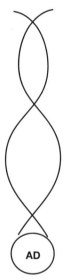

9q33-q34

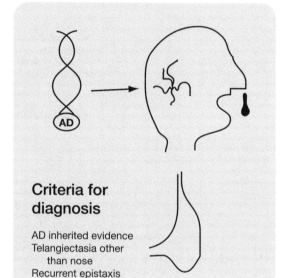

Criteria for diagnosis

AD inherited evidence
Telangiectasia other
   than nose
Recurrent epistaxis
Visceral involvement

Management

Epistaxis – oestrogen and
   embolisation
Cutaneous telangiectasia – lasers
Pulmonary AVM – embolise/ surgical
   resection
GI telangiectasia – oestrogen/
   progesterone tx
Brain AVM – surgery
Active bleeding – epsilon
   aminocaproic acid

Telangiectasia causes

Outdoor occupations
MS
Myxoedema
Pregnancy/ oestrogen
Scleroderma
Dermatomyositis
Acne rosacea
Lupus pernio

Hirsutism

= Male pattern hair growth in women due to
androgen sensitivity

Causes

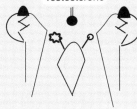

Testosterone

PCOS ○ (=an ovary)

Ovarian tumours ☆

CAH ◗ (=an adrenal on top of
a kidney)

Cushing's ◗

Prolactinoma ‖● (=a pituitary)

Androgen therapy Testosterone

Hair is abnormal, particularly on the upper
back, chin, chest and upper abdomen in
women

Investigations for PCOS
(mnemonic – piglet)

O varian USS
P rolactin elevation
G lucose
L H :FSH ratio raised >2:1
T estosterone

Treatment

Antiandrogens (spironolactone/ flutamide)
Finasteride
Shaving/ waxing, etc.

Hypopigmentation

Hypopigmentation differential

Hypopit
Albinism
Tuberous sclerosis
Phenylketonuria
Leprosy
Burns
Piebaldism

Hyperpigmentation differential (pimpled ass)

P BC
I ron overload
M alignancy
P orphyria cutanea tarda
L iver disease
E ndocrine (Addison's/ Cushing's, HiPTH)
D rugs (amiodarone/ 5FU/ bleomycin)

A rsenic
S cleroderma
S prue and malabsorption

Vitiligo

(= Loss of pigment-producing melanocytes in the epidermis. Main differential is pityriasis versicolor)

Associations (PaT AdDM)

Pa Pernicious anaemia
T hypoThyroidism/ hyperthyroidism
Ad Addison's
DM Diabetes mellitus

Also fibrosing alveolitis/ chronic autoimmune hepatitis/ alopecia areata

Management

>20% skin involved:
   Oral methoxsalen with PUVA
   Also: consider epidermal autografts and cultured epidermis
   Topical steroids/ skin bleaching

<20% skin involved:
   Methoxsalen with UVA then SPF15 sun cream

Reticulated Rashes

Erythema ab igne

(aka Granny's Tartan)

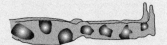

Benign reticulated rash usually over abdomen or front of legs. Related to application of heat

Livedo reticularis

Causes

PAN
SLE
Ca
Physiological
Atherosclerotic microemboli

Ichthyosis

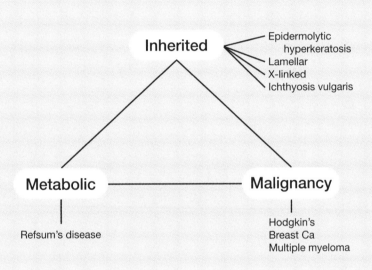

Inherited
— Epidermolytic
  hyperkeratosis
— Lamellar
— X-linked
— Ichthyosis vulgaris

Metabolic ——— Malignancy

Refsum's disease

Hodgkin's
Breast Ca
Multiple myeloma

Treatment: Regular emollients and moisturising creams (especially urea containing)

Legs

Causes of ulcers

Venous **O**
Arterial **O**
Vasculitis **⫽**
Haematological **●**

Cancer (BCC/ KS) **C**
Infection (fungal/
   syphilis) **I**
Trauma or artefact **T**

Venous ulcers ← → Arterial ulcers

Management

Decrease venous congestion
   with graduated compression
   bandages/ elevation
Infection (as for cellulitis)
Dermatitis: zinc in salicylic acid
Ulcers K permanganate/ skin
   graft/ debridement
Treatment for varicose veins

Features

Varicose veins
Haemosiderin deposition
   around ulcer
Surrounding dermatitis
Medial ulcer
Diagnosis via punch biopsy
   from border

Features

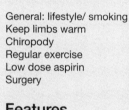

Management

General: lifestyle/ smoking
Keep limbs warm
Chiropody
Regular exercise
Low dose aspirin
Surgery

Features

Hairless skin
Cold
No peripheral pulses
Pale on elevation
Dependent rubor on dropping

Henoch–Schönlein Purpura

Features

Glomerulonephritis
Joint pains
Abdominal pain
Rash thigh and buttocks

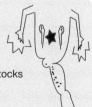

Investigation

Urine haematuria/
   proteinuria
ANA
VDRL
Skin biopsy

Treatment

If increased proteinuria,
   give steroids
Other treatments
   include ...
   plasma exchange
   IVIg
   cytotoxins

Malignant Melanoma

Types

Superficial spreading
Oval lentiginous
Mucous membrane
Lentigo maligna
    melanoma
Amelanotic
Miscellaneous

Predisposing factors

Freckles
Moles
Severe sunburn
Atypical naevi

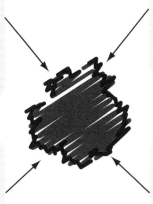

Features

Asymmetry
Border irregular
Colour variegation
Diameter >6mm

Prognosis

Tumour thickness
Level of invasion
Sex
Anatomical location

Treatment

Excision
Elective lymph node dissection in
    some cases
Interferon to prevent recurrence
Systemic chemotherapy if advanced

Miscellaneous Dermatology

Lichen simplex et chronicus

Management

Break the scratch-itch cycle
Topical steroids

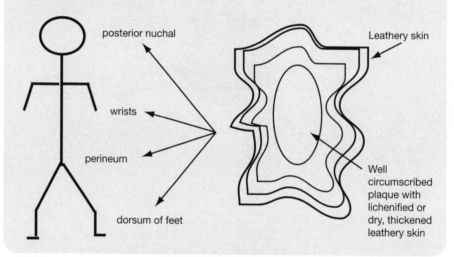

posterior nuchal

wrists

perineum

dorsum of feet

Leathery skin

Well circumscribed plaque with lichenified or dry, thickened leathery skin

Atopic dermatitis (=eczema)

Treatment

Avoid pruritogenic food
Avoid frequent baths
Adequate skin hydration
Treat infected skin
Antihistamines to control itching
Corticosteroid lotion, cream, ointment
Phototherapy with PUVA if unresponsive to topical treatment
Severe: ciclosporin/ azathioprine/ tacrolimus

Criteria for diagnosis (need 3 or more)

Pruritis
Flexure lichenification
Chronic/ relapsing dermatitis
Family or past history of atopy

Pigmented Lesions

Purpura

Causes

Medication (steroids/ thiazides/ sulphonylureas/ phenylbutazone)
Coagulation defects
Scurvy
Ehlers–Danlos' vasculitis

Acanthosis nigricans

Causes

Endocrine ...
Diabetes
Cushing's
Acromegaly
Stein–Leventhal syndrome

Cancer ...
Adenocarcinoma esp GI
Lymphoma

Pseudoxanthoma Elasticum

Angioid streaks (=abnormal elastic tissue in Bruch's retinal membrane)

If this is present 50% will have pseudoxanthoma
85% of pseudoxanthoma will have angioid streaks

Leopard skin spotting –
pathognomonic of pseudoxanthoma

Chicken skin appearance

CVS manifestations

MVP
Restrictive cardiomyopathy
Renovascular hypertension
CAD
PVD

GI manifestations

GI haemorrhage

Psoriasis

Genetics

Mostly polygenic
Some on chromosome 17

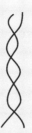

Things that make psoriasis worse

Drugs: antimalarials/ ACEI/ B-blockers/ COX-1 inhib

Infection: HIV/ beta haemolytic streps

Injury: mechanical/ sunburn

Type and distribution

Natural history

Type 1: Young with strong FH
Type 2: Old with no FH

Types of skin lesion
Chronic plaque
Guttate
Pustular
Erythrodermic

Severity score = PASI (Psoriasis Area and Severity Index)

Treatment

C alcipotriol/ coal tar (with PUVA B)
A nthracin
K eratolytics
E mollients (soft paraffin or aqueous cream)
S teroids (topical)

For refractory psoriasis

E tretinate
U ltraviolet A with methotrexate
S teroid (oral)
C iclosporin
U ltraviolet B
M ethotrexate alone

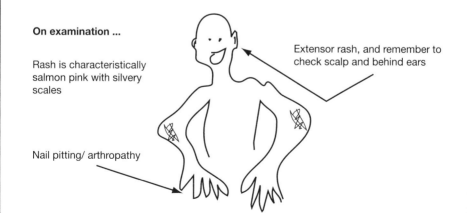

On examination ...

Rash is characteristically salmon pink with silvery scales

Extensor rash, and remember to check scalp and behind ears

Nail pitting/ arthropathy

Raynaud's Phenomenon

(Raynaud's disease if >3 yrs with no associated disease)

Causes

Immunological: SLE/MCTD/RA/scleroderma
Arterial: Atherosclerosis/thoracic outlet
Occupational: Vibration/cold
Drugs: B-blockers/ergot/sulphasalazine
Other: Cold agglutinins/cryoglobs/idiopathic

Investigations

IGs and electrophoresis/ANA
Routine bloods
Urine analysis
Chest and hand X-ray
Nail capillaroscopy

Treatment

Nitrates
Nifedipine
Prostaglandins
Dorsal sympathectomy

Other vasospastic conditions

Chilblains
Livedo reticularis
Erythromelalgia
White finger syndrome

Systemic Dermatological Manifestations 1

Erythema nodosum
A panniculitis – diagnosed on biopsy

Causes

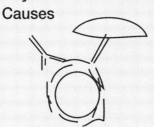

Sarcoidosis and TB ⟳ (=granulomas)
IBD and post-streptococcal infection ⟍ (=an antibody)
Drugs: Gold/ OCP/ Dapsone **GOD**
         Penicillin/ Aspirin/ Sulphonamide **PASS**
Fungal infections (yersinia/ histoplasmosis
   coccidioidomycosis)

GOD PASS

Treatment

Local: compression with heat/ cold
Systemic: NSAIDs/ KI/ steroids/ salicylates

Pyoderma gangrenosum

Causes

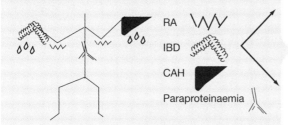

RA
IBD
CAH
Paraproteinaemia

Types

Peristomal (around a stoma)
Vulval
Penile
Pyostomatitis (in the mouth)
Associated with pre-leukaemia

Treatment

High dose steroids
Intralesional steroids
Dapsone
Dressings/ limb elevation

Erythema multiforme

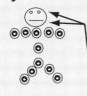

Target shaped lesions
  over limbs
Check hands and mouth
  for Stevens–Johnson
  bullae

Causes

Drugs (barbs/
  phenylbutazone/
  phenytoin)
Infections (HSV/ HIV/
  Mumps/ Hep B/
  Mycoplasma)
Sarcoid
Wegener's
SLE
Pregnancy
Malignancy

Tests

Viral titres
ASO titres
Mycoplasma
  serology

Management

IV fluids
Antibiotics
Steroids
Immunosuppressants
Aciclovir
Denudation of skin in
  burns unit

Systemic Dermatological Manifestations 2

Kaposi's sarcoma (HHV8 associated)

- **Classic:** Inactive. On the legs of elderly Jews
- **AIDS-associated:** Treat: Alpha-interferon + cytotoxic chemotherapy
- **African:** Aggressive. Associated with generalised lymphadenopathy
- **Transplantation:** Regress after therapy cessation

Management

Antiretrovirals
Interferon alpha
Intralesional chemotherapy
Systemic chemotherapy if aggressive
Radiation treatment
Surgery

Hairy leukoplakia

Causes

EBV in the context of AIDS

Treatment

Ganciclovir
Aciclovir

Molluscum contagiosum

Features: Small papular lesion with central punctum

Spread by autoinoculation

Pox virus

Squeezing   Curettage   Phenol ablation   Electrosurgery

Endocrinology

Acromegaly
Addison's Disease
Cushing's Syndrome
Exophthalmos
Graves' Disease
Gynaecomastia
Hypopituitarism
Hypothyroidism
Multinodular Goitre
Pretibial Myxoedema

Acromegaly

Questions regarding activity

Headache
Increased overall size
Sweatiness
Deterioration in vision

Tests

GH >2 ng/mL after OGTT
IGF-1
Pit function tests
Calcium – to exclude
    MEN1
MRI/perimetry

Treatment

Trans-sphenoidal surgery
Radiation
Octreotide and bromocriptine
Surgery gives immediate
    improvement in
    diaphoresis and carpal
    tunnel syndrome

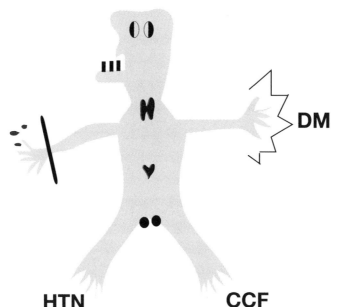

DM

HTN   **CCF**

Big hands

Carpal tunnel

Bitemporal hemianopia

Frontal bossing

Jaw jut and wide teeth

Arthropathy

Goitre

Sweaty

CCF/ DM/ HTN

Testicular atrophy

Addison's Disease

Causes

Acute

Sheehan's
PPAI
Trauma
Infection
Haemorrhage

Chronic

Autoimmune
TB/ HIV/ histoplasmosis
Amyloidosis/ sarcoid
Primary/ secondary
    cancer
Pit tumours
Steroid withdrawal

Associations

T hyroid (hypo and hyper)

O varian failure

P ernicious anaemia

Gland Polyglandular syndromes

Type 1:
Chronic mucocutaneous candidiasis
    hypoparathyroidism
Addison's

Type 2:
Addison's, IDDM, hypo/ hyperthyroidism

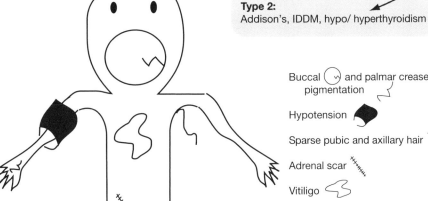

Buccal and palmar crease
    pigmentation

Hypotension

Sparse pubic and axillary hair

Adrenal scar

Vitiligo

Investigations

L   Lymphocytosis
E   Eosinophilia
U   Uraemia
C   Calcium   — All raised
K   Potassium
T   Hyperthyroid

Glucose decreased

Other tests

Short synacthen
ACTH and cortisol
    levels
Adrenal antibodies
CXR/ CT adrenals

Treatment

Prednisolone (5 mg am/
    2.5 mg pm)
Fludrocortisone
Steroid card
Medic Alert bracelet

Cushing's Syndrome

Cushing's disease = excess steroid from adrenals

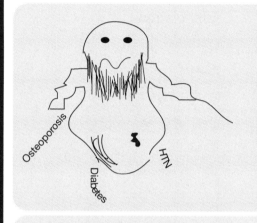

Features

Hirsutism
Proximal myopathy
Moon face
Truncal obesity
Striae
Easy bruising
Osteoporosis
Diabetes
Hypertension

Causes

Exogenous steroids
Ectopic
Pituitary adenoma
Adrenal ca/ adenoma

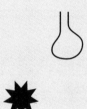

Investigations

24 hr urinary cortisol
Overnight dexamethasone
Plasma cortisol
High dose dexamethasone

Management

Surgical resection
Mitotane therapy
Trans-sphenoidal resection
Pituitary radiation
Surgical resection of tumour
CT/ MRI adrenals

Cushing's source

	Adrenal	Pituitary	Ectopic
ACTH	Dec	No change	Inc
High dose dex	No change in cortisol	Dec cortisol	No change in cortis
CRH stim	No change		
Metyrapone	Inc 11 deoxy <220	Inc 11 deoxycortisol >220	Inc 11 deoxy <220
Petrosal sinus ACTH	=Periph	>Periph	>Periph
	+USS abdo	+MRI gland	+CXR

Nelson's = Excess ACTH from non-suppressed pituitary post bilateral adrenalectomy

Exophthalmos

Eye signs

N o signs or symptoms
O nly lid retraction and stare

S oft tissue involved
P roptosis
E xtraocular muscles involved
C orneal involvement
S ight loss due to optic nerve
 involvement

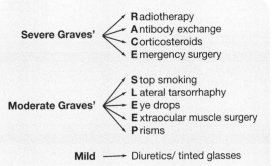

Severe Graves'
R adiotherapy
A ntibody exchange
C orticosteroids
E mergency surgery

Moderate Graves'
S top smoking
L ateral tarsorrhaphy
E ye drops
E xtraocular muscle surgery
P risms

Mild ⟶ Diuretics/ tinted glasses

NB: Radioiodine can make eye signs worse

Features of thyroid eye disease

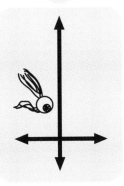

1. Proptosis – stand above patient's head

2. Dalrymple's sign – lid retraction – the sclera above
 the cornea will be seen

3. Lid lag – due to sympathetic overstimulation/ inferior
 rectus and levator myopathy

4. Extraocular muscles – ophthalmoplegia

5. Look for signs of thyrotoxicosis

Graves' Disease

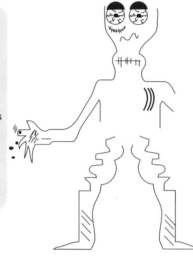

Causes of a hyperthyroid goitre

T hyroiditis
M ultinodular goitre
A utoimmune thyroiditis (=Graves')
N eoplasms (toxic adenoma)

Tests: T4/TSH/Thyroid autoantibodies

Lid lag
Proptosis
Tarsorraphy scars

Goitre
Thyroidectomy scar

Tremor
Atrial fib
Palmar erythema
Onycholysis
Sweatiness

Proximal myopathy
Tibial myxoedema

Treatment

Medications

Carbimazole/ methimazole/ propylthiouracil
 NB: High relapse rate also agranulocytosis/hepatitis

Radioactive iodine

Indications
M ultinodular goitre with CCF/AF
A utoimmune thyroiditis (Graves') with goitre and stable eye signs
N eoplasia, i.e. toxic adenoma

also ablation if severe CCF/AF/Ophthalmopathy/ psych problems

Contraindications
Breast feeding
Pregnancy
Allergy to iodine
Doesn't want catheter
and patient is incontinent

Advice
No pregnancy for 4–12 months
No contact for 12–28 days
Can get palpitations

Surgery indications

Large goitre
Patient preference
Drug non-compliance
Radioiodine not available

Isolated TSH suppression

Subclinical hyperthyroidism
Recovery from overt hyperthyroidism
Pregnancy in first trimester
Medications

Gynaecomastia

Physiological causes

Nausea
Adolescence
Ageing

Pathological causes

Liver disease
Klinefelter's
    syndrome
Viral orchitis
Renal failure
Neoplasm

Drugs

Antibiotics: isoniazid/
    ketoconazole/ metronidazole
CVS: atenolol/ captopril/ digoxin/
    enalapril/ methyldopa/
    nifedipine/ spironolactone/
    verapamil
Antiulcer: cimetidine/ ranitidine/
    omeprazole
Psychoactive: diazepam/ TCA

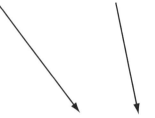

Investigations

CXR
Beta-hCG
LH and testosterone
PRL/ T3 and T4/TSH
Chromosome for Klinefelter's

Hypopituitarism

Features

Bitemporal hemianopia
Soft skin and crow's
     feet

Sparsity of hair

Breast tissue atrophy

Postural hypotension

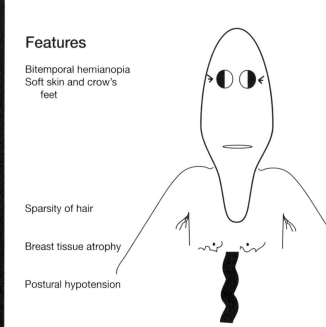

Causes

Post-partum pituitary
     necrosis
Cranial radiotherapy
Neurosarcoidosis
Any cause of a bitemporal
     hemianopia

Investigations

Perimetry
Skull X-ray
CT/ MRI
Pituitary stimulation test
     and hormone levels

Hypothyroidism

Cardiovascular

Bradycardia
HTN
Pericardial effusion
Inc LDL/ Dec HDL
Inc CK/ chol/ AST
Decreased Hb/ Na
CAD
CCF

Features

Coarse dry skin
Loss of outer third of eyebrows
Xanthelasma
Puffy eyelids
Thyroidectomy scar
Delayed tendon relaxation (single best
    indicator of hypothyroidism)
Constipation
Cold intolerance
Proximal myopathy

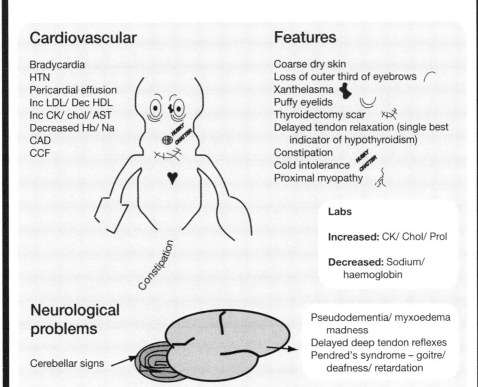

Labs

Increased: CK/ Chol/ Prol

Decreased: Sodium/
    haemoglobin

Neurological problems

Cerebellar signs

Pseudodementia/ myxoedema
    madness
Delayed deep tendon reflexes
Pendred's syndrome – goitre/
    deafness/ retardation

Causes of isolated raised TSH

Mild hypothyroidism
Amiodarone/ lithium
Recovery of hypothyroxinaemia from non-steroidal illness

Associations with Hashimoto's

Endo	Rheum	Haematol	Other
Addison's	RA	PA	UC
DM	SLE	H anaemia	Ovarian failure
Dec PTH	Sjögren's		
Graves'			

Multinodular Goitre

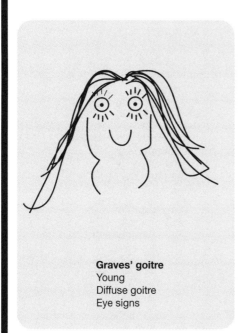

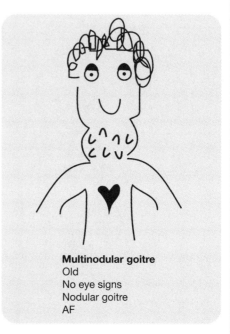

Graves' goitre
Young
Diffuse goitre
Eye signs

Multinodular goitre
Old
No eye signs
Nodular goitre
AF

Investigation

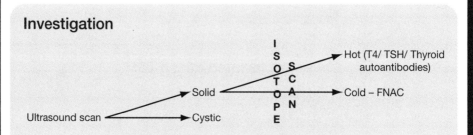

Ultrasound scan → Solid → ISOTOPE SCAN → Hot (T4/ TSH/ Thyroid autoantibodies)

Ultrasound scan → Cystic

Solid → Cold – FNAC

Treatment

1. Toxic
Beta-blockade +/– warfarin
(if AF)
Surgery
Radioiodine

2. Non-toxic
Thyroxine
Surgery
Radioiodine

Pretibial Myxoedema

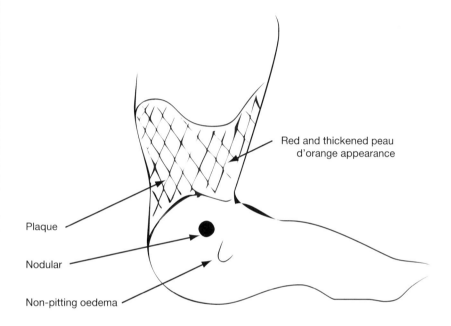

Red and thickened peau d'orange appearance

Plaque

Nodular

Non-pitting oedema

Also

Elephantiasis form
Polypoid form

Treatment

S teroids (intralesional)
O ctreotide
C ytotoxins
A ntibody exchange

Ophthalmology

Cataracts

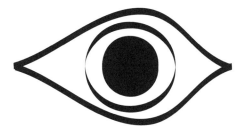

Black silhouette against red of retina

Causes

Old age
Diabetes
Metabolic: Cushing's/ Wilson's/ hypoparathyroidism
Infection: congenital CMV/ rubella
Myotonic dystrophy
Drugs: steroids/ chloroquine

Diabetic Retinopathy

Background retinopathy

After 20 years of Type 1 DM, most patients will have some of these

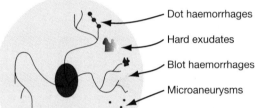

- Dot haemorrhages
- Hard exudates
- Blot haemorrhages
- Microaneurysms

Preproliferative retinopathy

- Venous beading
- Cotton wool spots
- Large deep haemorrhages

Maculopathy

Circinate oedema with macula at its centre

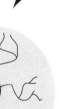

Proliferative retinopathy

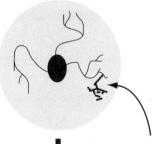

Vitreous haemorrhage and new, fragile vessel formation

Management

Keep diabetes under control
Refer to ophthalmologist

Maculopathy and proliferative retinopathy are treatable by laser photocoagulation

Other points

1 in 3 diabetics will develop eye problems
After 30 years of diabetes 5% will become blind
This is related to poor glycaemic control, smoking and hypertension

Rubeosis iridis

Hypertensive Retinopathy

Stages

1. Silver wiring

2. Nipping

3. Haemorrhage/ cotton wool spots

4. Papilloedema (associated with end-organ damage and increased mortality)

Cotton wool spots differential

HIV infection
Anaemia
Infective endocarditis
Leukaemia
Diabetic retinopathy

Miscellaneous Ophthalmology 1

Age-related macular degeneration

Drusen

(=Material between Bruch's
   membrane and pigment
   epithelium. Very common in
   elderly. Only a risk if large)

Choroidal neovascularisation

Find on fluorescein angiography/
   retinal angiography
Treat with photocoagulation/
   surgery/ radiotherapy/
   thalidomide

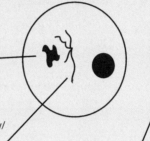

Central scotoma

Old chorioretinitis

White areas of choroidal
   atrophy with pigmented edges

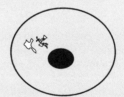

Causes

Sarcoidosis
Syphilis
TB
Behcet's
Toxoplasmosis
CMV
AIDS

Vitreous opacities

Features

White opacities in front of
   retinal vessels
Can cause monocular diplopia

Causes

Blood
Cholesterol bulbi
Asteroid hyalosis

Monocular diplopia causes

Opacities in lens
Corneal opacities
Retinal detachment

Miscellaneous Ophthalmology 2

Retinal AIDS

CMV retinitis

'Pizza pie fundus'

Treatment

Foscarnet + antiretroviral
or
ganciclovir (with impaired renal function)

Retinal detachment

Features

Opaque retina
Folds appear when a
lot of sub-retinal
fluid present

Types

Rhegmatogenous – break in retina that
allows fluid in. Trauma related. Fix with
scleral buckling procedure

Traction – traction from contracting retinal
membranes. Treated with pars plana
vitrectomy

Secondary – due to systemic disorders
such as glomerulonephritis/ retinal
vasculitis, etc.

Subhyaloid haemorrhage

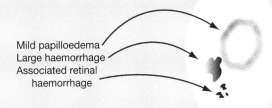

Mild papilloedema
Large haemorrhage
Associated retinal
haemorrhage

Optic Atrophy

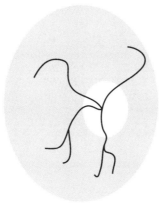

Clearly delineated and pale disc margin

Central scotoma

Causes

Demyelinating disease
Optic nerve compression
Glaucoma

Ischaemia
Nutritional amblyopia (e.g. B12 deficiency)
Toxic amblyopia (quinine, lead, arsenic)
Hereditary (Leber's optic atrophy, Friedreich's
    ataxia)

Papilloedema

Causes

**Any cause of raised
 intracranial pressure**

Metabolic causes
CO2 retention
Steroid withdrawal
Thyroid eye disease
Vitamin A intoxication
Lead poisoning

Increased protein in CSF
Guillain–Barré
Spinal cord tumour/ block

Haematological problems
Superior vena cava
 obstruction
Central retinal vein occlusion
Polycythaemia rubra vera
Multiple myeloma

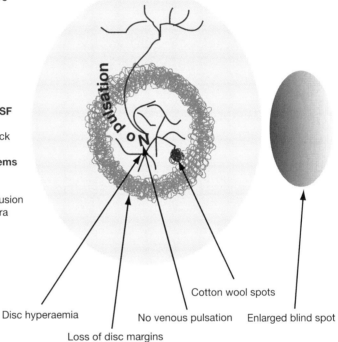

Cotton wool spots

Disc hyperaemia

No venous pulsation

Enlarged blind spot

Loss of disc margins

Stages of papilloedema

I   Venous calibre and tortuosity
II Pink cup. Vessels disappear suddenly
III Disc blurring
IV Suffusion of whole disc

Retinitis Pigmentosa

Features

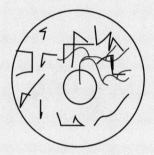

Night blindness and tunnel vision

Pale optic disc

Bone spicules

Pigmentation hides the course of the vessels (in chorioretinitis, the vessels go anterior)

Systemic associations (ALURK)

Abetalipoproteinaemia

Malabsorption
Abetalipoproteinaemia
Acanthocytosis
Spinocerebellar disease

Kearn–Sayre syndrome

Heart block
Progressive external ophthalmoplegia

Laurence–Moon–Biedl (AR)

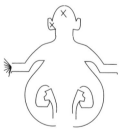

Retardation
Polydactyly
Renal cystic disease
Deafness

Usher's syndrome

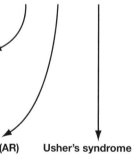

Bilateral deafness

Refsum's disease

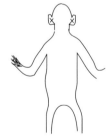

Peripheral neuropathy
Deafness
Cerebellar ataxia
Ichthyosis

Retinal Vein and Artery Occlusion

Retinal vein occlusion

Causes

Central (C) or Branch (B)

HTN
DM
Raised ICP
Hyperviscosity
Vasculitides

CRVO
BRVO

Haemorrhages (blood and
    thunder)
Cotton wool spots
Neovascularisation
Vascular sheathing
Loss of vision – sudden
Relative afferent pupillary
    defect if severe occlusion

Treatment

Regular ophthalmological follow-up as
    neovascularisation may need laser treatment

Complications

Retinal neovascularisation
Rubeosis iridis
Rubeotic glaucoma

Retinal artery occlusion

Increased ICP
Embolism
GCA
Sickle cell
Cocaine
Syphilis

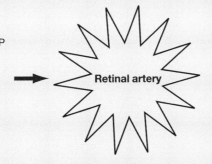

Retinal artery

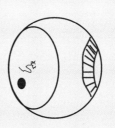

?

Treatment

Supine position
Ocular massage
Acetazolamide
5% CO_2 and 95% O_2 inhalation
Anterior chamber paracentesis

Miscellaneous

Achondroplasia
Chronic Lymphocytic Leukaemia
Clubbing
Down's Syndrome
Dupuytren's Contracture
Ehlers–Danlos' Syndrome
Klinefelter's Syndrome
Marfan's Syndrome
Miscellaneous
Osteoporosis
Paget's Disease
Peutz–Jeghers' Syndrome
Tuberous Sclerosis
Turner's Syndrome

Achondroplasia

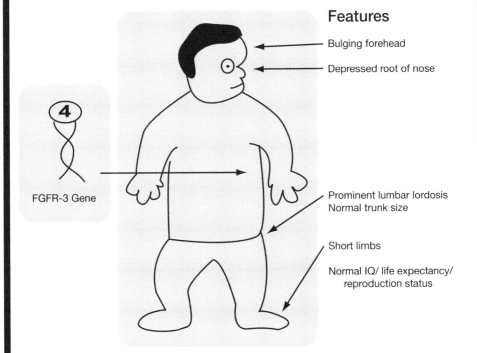

Features

Bulging forehead

Depressed root of nose

FGFR-3 Gene

Prominent lumbar lordosis
Normal trunk size

Short limbs

Normal IQ/ life expectancy/
reproduction status

Complications

Hydrocephalus
Compression of brainstem/ cord/ roots

Chronic Lymphocytic Leukaemia

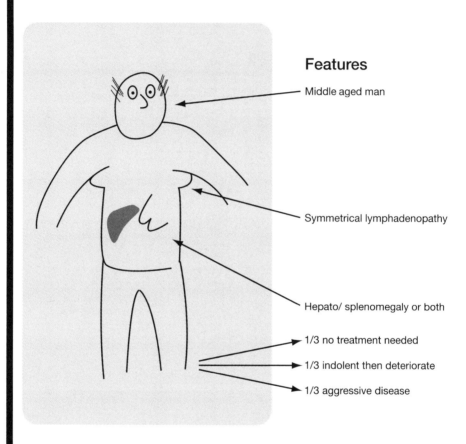

Features

Middle aged man

Symmetrical lymphadenopathy

Hepato/ splenomegaly or both

1/3 no treatment needed

1/3 indolent then deteriorate

1/3 aggressive disease

Staging

a. No anaemia or thrombocytopenia and <3 lymph nodes
b. As A but >3 lymph nodes
c. Anaemia or thrombocytopenia

Treatment

Consider steroids/ chlorambucil/ fludarabine

Clubbing

Grades

I Glossy and cyanotic skin

II Nail bed angle obliterated

III Drum-stick appearance

IV Bony changes

Causes

Respiratory
Asbestosis
Bronchiectasis
Cryptogenic fibrosing alveolitis
Cancer
Chronic suppurative lung disease
Ext allergic alveolitis
Mesothelioma

Abdo
Coeliac/ Whipple's
Polyposis coli
IBD
Cirrhosis

CVS
Infective endocarditis
Congenital cyanotic heart disease

Down's Syndrome

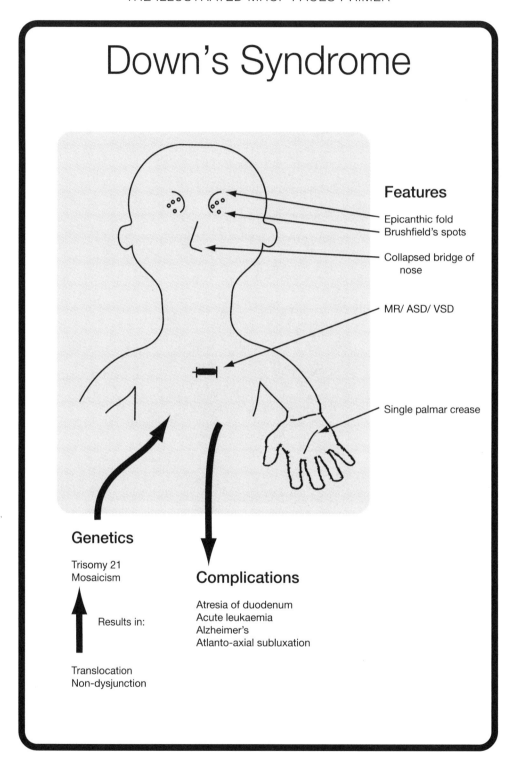

Features

Epicanthic fold
Brushfield's spots

Collapsed bridge of
nose

MR/ ASD/ VSD

Single palmar crease

Genetics

Trisomy 21
Mosaicism

Results in:

Translocation
Non-dysjunction

Complications

Atresia of duodenum
Acute leukaemia
Alzheimer's
Atlanto-axial subluxation

Dupuytren's Contracture

Features

Thickened palmar fascia

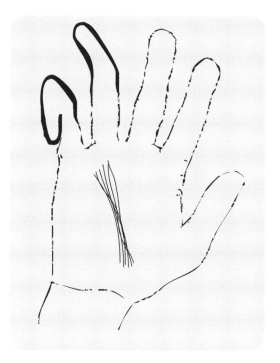

Associations

Alcoholism
Antiepileptics
Peyronie's disease
Retroperitoneal fibrosis
Chronic systemic problems (diabetes mellitus/
    TB/ cirrhosis)

Treatment

Triamcinolone
Surgery

Ehlers–Danlos' Syndrome

A collagen synthesis disorder

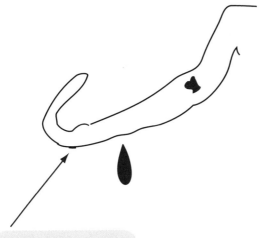

Complications

CVS:
MVP/ dissection

Abdominal:
Megacolon
Achalasia
Hernia
Eventration of diaphragm

Diagnostic criteria

Fragile skin
Bleeding diathesis
Hypermobile joints

9 point score for hypermobility based on ...

Hyperextended elbow >10°
Hyperextended knee >10°
Apposition of thumb to volar aspect of forearm
Hyperextension of fifth MCP joint to 90°

Klinefelter's Syndrome

Usually 47XXY chromosomal abnormality

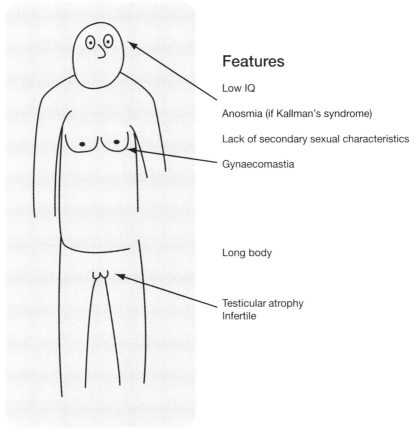

Features

Low IQ

Anosmia (if Kallman's syndrome)

Lack of secondary sexual characteristics

Gynaecomastia

Long body

Testicular atrophy
Infertile

Investigations

Chromosomal analysis
Reduced testosterone
Raised FSH
Oestradiol

Marfan's Syndrome

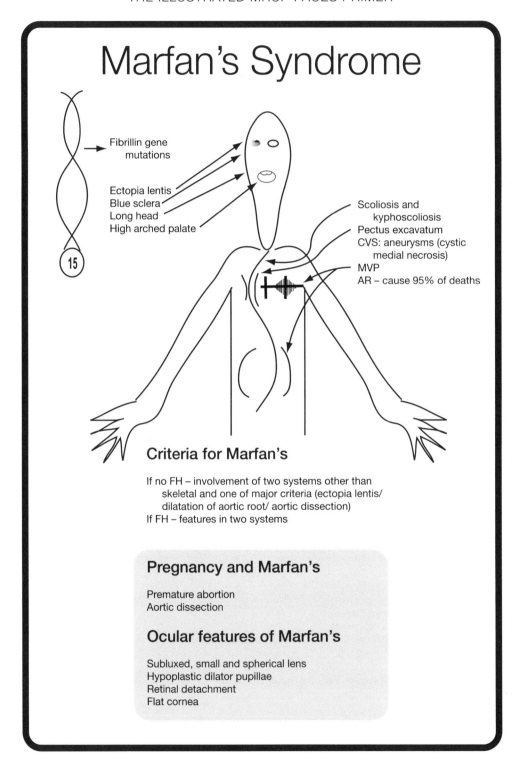

Fibrillin gene
    mutations

Ectopia lentis
Blue sclera
Long head
High arched palate

15

Scoliosis and
    kyphoscoliosis
Pectus excavatum
CVS: aneurysms (cystic
    medial necrosis)
MVP
AR – cause 95% of deaths

Criteria for Marfan's

If no FH – involvement of two systems other than
    skeletal and one of major criteria (ectopia lentis/
    dilatation of aortic root/ aortic dissection)
If FH – features in two systems

Pregnancy and Marfan's

Premature abortion
Aortic dissection

Ocular features of Marfan's

Subluxed, small and spherical lens
Hypoplastic dilator pupillae
Retinal detachment
Flat cornea

Miscellaneous

Macroglossia

True macroglossia 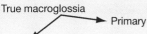 → Primary

Secondary – amyloidosis/ acromegaly/ angioedema/ lymphoma/ chronic infection/ SOL

Pseudomacroglossia – small mandible, e.g. Down's/ Pierre–Robin/ cerebral palsy

Complications – breathing/ eating/ ulcers

The diabetic foot

Neuropathic foot	**Ischaemic foot**
Pink and warm	Cold
Plantar ulcer	Pulseless
Decreased light touch, peripheral and vibration sensation	Shiny
	Ulcers on heels and toes

Parotid enlargement

Causes of painless bilateral parotid enlargement

Sarcoidosis
Sjögren's/ keratoconjunctivitis sicca
Lymphoma/ leukaemia

Obesity

Always enquire regarding
BP
DM   BMI = kg/m² (NR = 18.5–25)
Lipids
BMI
Osteoarthritis and sleep apnoea
Rule out family history and secondary causes

Treatment

Multidisciplinary/ drugs/ surgery (gastric bypass/ banding)

Lymphadenopathy

Causes

Viral – EBV/ CMV/ HIV
Bact – TB/ syphilis/ brucellosis
Haem – lymphoma/ CLL/ ALL
Rheum – SLE/ RA/ sarcoid
Drugs – phenytoin

Osteogenesis imperfecta

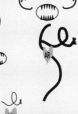

Otosclerosis and hearing loss
Old fractures
Defective dentine formation
Kyphosis and scoliosis
Joint hypermobility
Aortic regurgitation

SVC obstruction

Causes

Cancer
Lymphoma
Aortic aneurysm
Mediastinal goitre
Mediastinal fibrosis
Constrictive pericarditis

Management

IV frusemide
Chemotherapy
Mediastinal irradiation
Stents
Mechanical thrombectomy

Gingival hypertrophy

Causes

Phenytoin
Ciclosporin
Leukaemia

Glass eye

Causes

Trauma
Malignant melanoma

Osteoporosis

Features

Usually woman
Kyphosis
Protuberant abdomen

Investigations

Myeloma screen
Testosterone in men
Thyroid function tests
DEXA scan

Treatment

Lifestyle changes
Oestrogen treatment
Calcium and vitamin D
Alendronate/ strontium
Calcitonin nasal spray

Primary causes

Type 1 Vertebral and Colles' fractures. Due to oestrogen deficiency

Type 2 Proximal femur. Due to age-related bone loss.

Secondary causes

Long secondary amenorrhoea
Primary hypogonadism
Steroids
Anorexia
Primary hyperparathyroidism
Chronic renal failure
Hyperthyroidism
Immobility
Smoking
Alcohol
Underweight

Paget's Disease

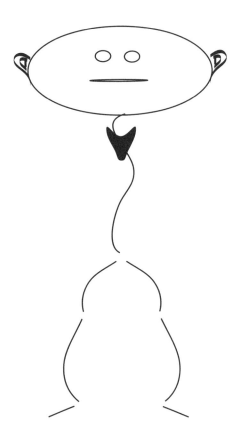

8th nerve compression
(sensorineural deafness) or
malformed ossicle
(conductive deafness)
Large skull diameter (>55 mm)
Optic atrophy

Signs of CCF

Kyphosis

Vertebral bruits

Anterior tibial bowing

Lateral femoral bowing

Complications: Fractures/ cord compression/ osteosarcomas/ CCF
Labs: Raised alk phos/ raised 24 hr urinary hydroxyproline
Treatment: Bisphosphonate/ calcitonin/ surgery

Peutz–Jeghers' Syndrome

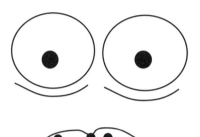

Features

Freckles over lips and mouth
Looks anaemic
Hamartomatous polyps

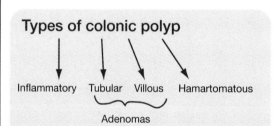

Types of colonic polyp

Inflammatory   Tubular   Villous   Hamartomatous

Adenomas

Polyposis syndromes

FAP
Gardner's
Turcot's
Familial juvenile polyposis
Cowden's
Peutz–Jeghers'

Tuberous Sclerosis

Features

Retinal glial hamartomas

Adenoma sebaceum

Ash leaf macules

Subungual fibromas

Shagreen patches
(over back)

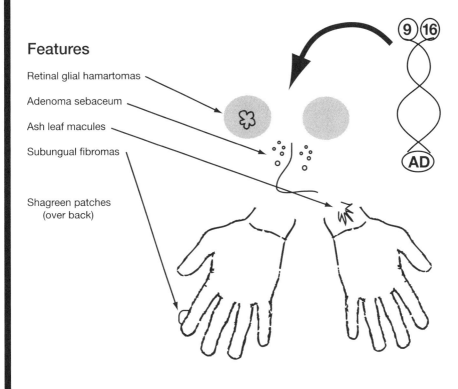

Associations

CNS hamartomas
Renal angiomyolipomas
Cardiac rhabdomyomas
Cysts liver/ kidney

3rd Nerve Palsy

Causes

D iabetes

V ascular < Hypertension
Aneurysm

D emyelination

T rauma
I nfection (encephalitis)
C ancer (base of skull/
meningioma)
S yphilis

+ophthalmoplegic migraine

Presentation

Unilateral ptosis
Dilated pupil
Accommodation and light paralysis
Eye is down and out

NB: Suspect 3rd nerve nucleus lesion if
bilateral 3rd nerve palsy or unilat 3rd
with contralat 6th

Tests

BP
Glucose
ESR
TFTs
Edrophonium
CT scan

6th Nerve Palsy

Causes

D iabetes

V ascular < Hypertension
Aneurysm

D emyelination

T rauma
I nfection (encephalitis)
C ancer (nasopharyngeal
cancer and acoustic
neuroma)
S yphilis

+increased ICP

Anatomy

Superior optic foramen

Midbrain

Pons

V VII

MLF PRF

Medulla

Cavernous
sinus

Presentation

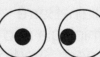

Failure to abduct eye (in this case right)

7th Nerve Palsy

Anatomy

Lesion localisation

Nuclei in the pons – assoc 6th nerve palsy
Cerebellopontine angle lesion – 5th and 8th
    involved
Bony canal – loss of taste and hyperacusis
Forehead spared in upper motor neurone
    7th nerve palsy

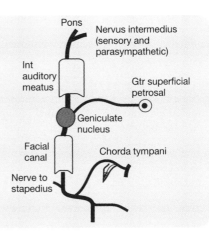

Pons

Nervus intermedius
(sensory and
parasympathetic)

Int
auditory
meatus

Gtr superficial
petrosal

Geniculate
nucleus

Facial
canal

Chorda tympani

Nerve to
stapedius

Unilateral facial nerve palsy

UMN

Stroke

LMN

1. Idiopathic (Bell's)
2. Herpes zoster
3. Cerebellopontine angle tumour
4. Parotid tumours
5. Old polio
6. Otitis media
7. Skull fracture

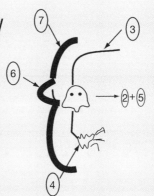

Bilateral facial nerve palsy

Causes

= sarcoid/ GB/ Lyme and the 3 Ms

Sarcoidosis
Guillain–Barré
Lyme disease
Myasthenia gravis
Muscular dystrophy
Motor neurone disease

Treatment

Physio/ eye protection
Aciclovir
Prednisolone

Argyll Robertson Pupil

Causes

Diabetes
Vascular
Demyelination
Trauma
Infection (Lyme/ encephalitis)
Cancer
Syphilis/ sarcoid

The light reflex

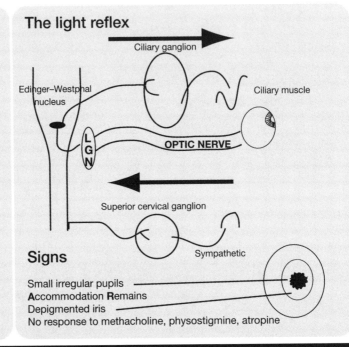

Ciliary ganglion
Edinger–Westphal nucleus
Ciliary muscle
OPTIC NERVE
L G N
Superior cervical ganglion
Sympathetic

Signs

Small irregular pupils
Accommodation **R**emains
Depigmented iris
No response to methacholine, physostigmine, atropine

Holmes–Adie Syndrome

= Adie's tonic pupil and absent deep tendon jerks

Causes of a dilated pupil

Mydriatic eye drops
3rd nerve palsy
Holmes–Adie pupil

Causes of a small pupil

Old age
Pilocarpine eye drops
Horner's
Argyll Robertson
Pontine lesions
Narcotics

Pathology

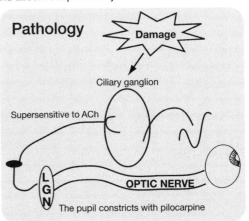

Damage
Ciliary ganglion
Supersensitive to ACh
OPTIC NERVE
L G N
The pupil constricts with pilocarpine

Becker's and Other Muscular Dystrophies

Becker's muscular dystrophy

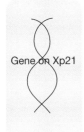

Gene on Xp21

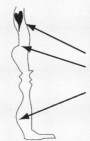

Features

Young adult male >15 yrs
Cardiomyopathy
Kyphoscoliosis
Low IQ
Pseudohypertrophy of calves

Diagnosis

Muscle biopsy and Western blot stain showing decreased/ abnormal dystrophin

Fascioscapulohumeral dystrophy

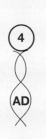

4

AD

Features

Ptosis
Expressionless face
Wasted sternocleidomastoid
Winged scapula ⟶
Weak biceps/ triceps
Absent biceps/ triceps reflexes

Winged scapula

If on its own, is due to palsy of the long thoracic nerve of Bell which supplies serratus anterior, or trapezius paralysis

Limb girdle dystrophy

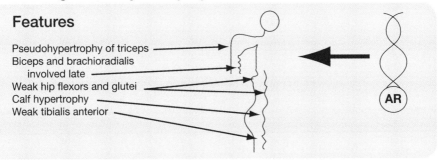

Features

Pseudohypertrophy of triceps
Biceps and brachioradialis involved late
Weak hip flexors and glutei
Calf hypertrophy
Weak tibialis anterior

AR

Bilateral Spastic Paralysis (Spastic Paraparesis)

Causes

Adults
Friedreich's ataxia
SACD
Tabes dorsalis

Transverse myelitis
Heredity spastic paraplegia
Tropical spastic paraplegia

Spinal cord tumour
Syringomyelia
Trauma

Elderly
OA cervical spine
Vitamin deficiency
Mets
Ant spinal artery thrombosis
Spinal cord vasc atherosclerosis

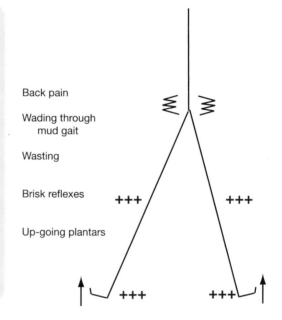

Back pain

Wading through
    mud gait

Wasting

Brisk reflexes   +++   +++

Up-going plantars

+++   +++

Investigation

Serum B12/ PSA/ protein
    electrophoresis
MRI/ CT
CSF for oligoclonal bands

Brown–Séquard Syndrome

Hemisection of the spinal cord

Causes

Any cord compression
Syringomyelia
Cord tumour
Haematomyelia
Bullet/ stab wounds

Features

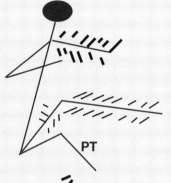

PT

Ipsilateral mono/ hemiplegia
Ipsilateral loss of joint position and vibration
Contralateral loss of pain and temperature sensation

Cauda Equina Syndrome

Causes

Disc/ spondylolisthesis
Tumours

Features

Pain ant thigh
Wasted quads
Weak foot inverters
Absent knee jerk

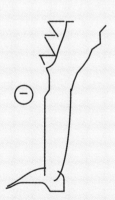

Carpal Tunnel Syndrome

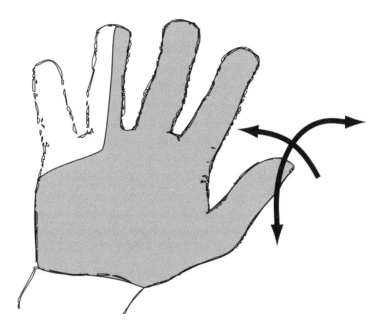

Causes

OCP
Steroids
RA
Myxoedema
Acromegaly
Sarcoidosis
Hyperparathyroid

Treatment

Diuretics
Wrist splint
Local steroids
Surgical decompression

Features

Decreased sensation over
   the palm and radial 3½ fingers
Weak flexion, abduction and
   opposition of the thumb
Tinnel's sign

Cerebellar Syndrome

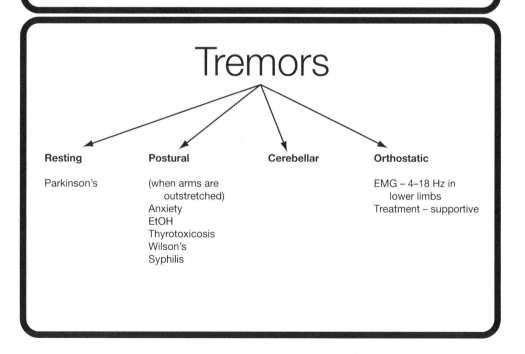

Causes

Tumours
Vascular
Hypothyroid (T)
EtOH (E)
Phenytoin (A for
    antiepileptics)
MS (M)
Paraneoplastic
Friedreich's
    ataxia

Friedreich's

TEAM

Localise the lesion
cerebellar signs

Clinical

D ysdiadochokinesis
A taxia
N ystagmus (towards side
    of lesion)
I ntention tremor
S lurred speech (usually
    bilateral lesion)
H ypotonia

Posterior lobe (=truncal ataxia) **Lateral lobe** (=limb ataxia) **Anterior lobe** (=gait ataxia)

Tremors

Resting	**Postural**	**Cerebellar**	**Orthostatic**
Parkinson's	(when arms are outstretched) Anxiety EtOH Thyrotoxicosis Wilson's Syphilis		EMG – 4–18 Hz in lower limbs Treatment – supportive

Charcot–Marie–Tooth Disease

(= Peroneal Muscular Atrophy)

Features

Inverted champagne bottle
    legs
Lateral popliteal nerve
    thickening
Achilles contracture
Pes cavus
Absent ankle jerk
Sometimes stocking sensory
    loss
Claw toes
High stepping gait

Types

17 or 1 or X

AD or AR

HSMN I – demyelinating neuropathy
HSMN II – axonal neuropathy
Distal spinal muscular atrophy

Other hereditary neuropathies

Fabry's
Tangier
Refsum's
Roussy–Lévy
Bassen–Kornzweig
Metachromatic leukodystrophy

Chorea

Quasipurposive, dynamic movement

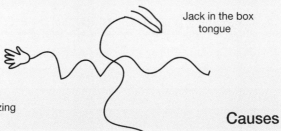

Jack in the box tongue

Milkmaid's grip (squeezing and relaxing)

Causes

SLE
Polycythaemia
Pregnancy
Hypoparathyroidism
CVA
Acanthocytosis
Huntington's

Hemiballismus

Usually CVA – ipsilat subthalamic nucleus of Luys

Treatment: haloperidol/ tetrabenazine/ thalamotomy/ pallidectomy

Combined Cranial Nerve Problems

Cerebellopontine angle tumour

The angle is defined by a triangle of the cerebellum, lateral pons and inner third of the petrous temporal bone

Causes

Medulloblastoma/
   meningioma
Astrocytoma
Cholesteatoma
Haemangioma
Acoustic neuroma
Glioma
+Syphilis/ TB/ basilar
   artery aneurysm

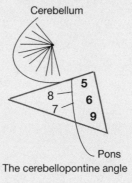

Cerebellum

Pons

The cerebellopontine angle

Tests

Head CT/ LP
Audiogram/ caloric
VDRL

Treatment

Microsurgical resection
Stereotactic radiosurgery
Conservative

Jugular foramen syndrome

Causes

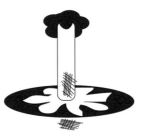

Carcinoma of the pharynx
Fractured base of skull
Paget's
Basal meningitis
Neurofibroma
Thrombosis of jugular vein

Features

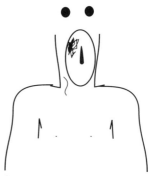

Sluggish palatal movement
Absent gag reflex on the same
   side
Wasted sternomastoid

Deformed Lower Limb

Causes: **Spina bifida**   **Old poliomyelitis**

Spina bifida

Bony changes on X-ray –
     scoliosis, erosions and
     spurs

Hypertrichosis/ naevus/
     scarring/ lipoma/ dimple

Unilateral short leg and
     deficient muscles below
     the knee

Sensory loss L5/ S1

Prenatal screening tests

Amniotic alpha fetoprotein
High res USS
Amniotic ACh estimation

Polio

Prevention

Sabin (live) ⟶ Causes
Salk (killed)   vaccine-associated
van Wezel   paralytic
   (enhanced)   poliomyelitis (VAPA)

Types
(picornaviridae)

I   Brunhilde
II   Lansing
III Leon

Causes of LMN signs in the legs

Peripheral neuropathy
Prolapsed intervertebral disc
Diabetic amyotrophy
Poliomyelitis
Cauda equina lesion
Motor neurone disease
Peroneal muscular atrophy

Dystrophia Myotonica

myotonia = continued contraction after voluntary contraction has ceased,
followed by impaired relaxation

Genes

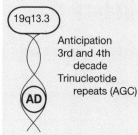

19q13.3

Anticipation
3rd and 4th
decade
Trinucleotide
repeats (AGC)

AD

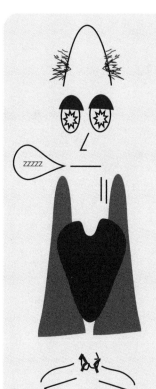

Features

Frontal balding with
smooth forehead

Bilateral ptosis
Stellate cataracts

Expressionless face
Somnolence

Wasted masseter and
sternocleidomastoid

Dysphagia

Cardiomyopathy and
conduction defects

Respiratory infections
(low serum IgG)

Testicular atrophy

Distal muscle weakness
and myotonia

Depressed deep tendon
jerks

Also ... gynaecomastia
and diabetes mellitus

Genetic screening and diagnosis

EMG (dive bomber pattern)
Slit lamp (cataracts)
Some pre-natal diagnosis possible

Treatment

Phenytoin if disabling myotonia
Foot drop – calipers
Heart block – pacemaker
Myotonia Society

Friedreich's Ataxia

Genes

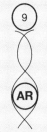

9

AR

Features

Cerebellar signs 🎻 ↔

Kyphoscoliosis ∫

Optic atrophy

Posterior and lateral
degeneration
Peripheral sensory
nerve fibre
degeneration
Posterior root
ganglion loss

Absent knee jerks
Distal muscle wasting
Pes cavus
Position and vibration
sense loss (VP-ve
on diagram)
Upgoing plantars

20 yrs to RIP

VP ⊖

Diagnostic criteria

Harding's criteria
Onset before age of 25
Absent knee and absent ankle jerks
Extensor plantars
AR inheritance
Motor conduction abnormalities >40 ms
Small or absent sensory nerve potentials

Associations

Cardiomyopathy
Optic and retinal atrophy
Diabetes mellitus
Mild dementia

Other causes of spinocerebellar disease

Roussy–Lévy disease (lower limb atrophy
and areflexia)
Refsum's disease
Bassen–Kornzweig disease (vitamin E
deficiency)
Olivopontocerebellar degeneration (CAG
repeat – chromosome 6)
Machado–Joseph
Dentatorubral pallidoluysian atrophy

Causes of absent knee and upgoing plantars

Peripheral neuropathy in a stroke patient
MND
Conus medullaris
Tabes dorsalis
SACD
Friedreich's ataxia

Gait

Cerebellar gait (see cerebellar syndrome)

Parkinsonian gait (see Parkinson's)

Hemiplegic gait (see hemiplegia)

Foot stomping = sensory ataxia

High stepping gait = foot drop

Foot drop

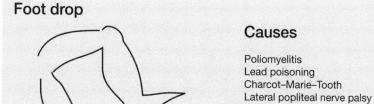

Causes

Poliomyelitis
Lead poisoning
Charcot–Marie–Tooth
Lateral popliteal nerve palsy

Features

Foot dorsiflexion and eversion weakness
Lateral calf wasting
High stepping
Sensation loss on lateral leg and dorsum of foot

Scissor gait = spastic paraparesis

Waddling gait = proximal myopathy

Marche a petit pas = normal pressure hydrocephalus

Guillain–Barré

A demyelinating neuropathy

Features

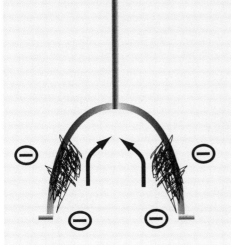

Ascending demyelinating polyneuropathy

Distal weakness and sensory loss
Areflexia

Tests

Nerve conduction studies – conduction
    block
Albumino-cytological dissociation (CSF)
Spirometry and BP

Treatment

High dose IV Ig
Physio
Ventilation

Hemiplegia and Strokes

TACS – Total anterior circulation stroke

Homonymous hemianopia
Unilateral sensory deficit face/arm/leg
Higher cerebral function problems

PACS – Partial anterior circulation stroke

= 2 of the 3 features of TACS

Lacunar

Pure motor: unilateral 2 of face/ arm/ leg
Pure sensory: "   "
Ataxic hemiparesis: ipsilat cerebellar and corticospinal

Sensorimotor: unilateral pure sensory and pure motor combined

POCI – Posterior circulation infarct

Bilateral motor/ sensory signs
Cerebellar signs
Diplopia +/– palsy of eye
Crossed signs
Hemianopia

Cerebellar sign

Investigations and treatment

Stop smoking
Aspirin
Carotid artery DSA
Consider thrombolysis in acute stage
Carotid duplex

Carotid endarterectomy
70–99% stenosis – risk <benefit
30–69% stenosis – still being evaluated
0–29% stenosis – benefit >risk

TIAs

Carotid

Acute loss of focal cerebral or ocular function with symptoms <24 hours

Aphasia
Hemiparesis
Amaurosis fugax

1/6 will have a CVA in 5 years
1/4 will die in 5 years

Vertebrobasilar TIA

Drop attack/ vertigo/ dysphagia
Sudden bilateral blindness
Bilateral alternating sensory weakness

Stroke outcome measures

HTN Smoking AF DM
Bruit Lipidaemia IHD High haematocrit
PVD OCP Cardiomyopathy
TIA

Stroke outcome measures

Barthel – ADLs
Rankin – overall function
Glasgow outcome – overall function
NHS stroke – neurological deficit

Other causes of a hemiparesis

In the elderly	In the young	Investigations and treatment
Vascular	I nfection	ESR/ glucose
Tumour	N eoplasia	ECHO/ DSA
Subdural	S yphilis	
Syphilis	T rauma	
	E mboli	Physio and stop
	A utoimmune	risk factors
	M S	

Horner's Syndrome

(Miosis + ptosis + anhydrosis + enophthalmos)

Causes

Neck surgery/ trauma
Carotid/ aortic aneurysms
Brainstem vascular lesion
Pancoast's
Cervical LN
Idiopathic
Brainstem demyelination

How to examine a Horner's patient

1. Hands
   Wasting (Pancoast's)
   Clubbing
2. Neck
   Cervical
      sympathectomy scar
   Lymph nodes
   Pancoast's dullness
   Carotid aneurysm
3. Look for evidence of
      demyelination

Central vs peripheral causes

Central causes
Demyelination
Vascular lesions
Syringomyelia

Peripheral causes
Cervical LN
Pancoast's
Carotid and aortic
   lesions
Neck surgery

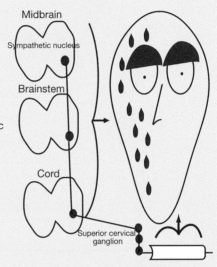

	Central lesions	Peripheral lesions
Cocaine 4% in both eyes:	Dilates both	Dilates normal eye only
Adrenaline 1:1000 both eyes:	No effect bilaterally	Dilates affected only

Ptosis

Causes of a unilateral ptosis

3 rd nerve palsy
H orner's
I diopathic/ congen
M yasthenia gravis

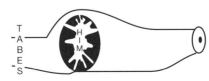

T
A
B
E
S

Causes of a bilateral ptosis

Dystrophia myotonica
Ocular myopathy
Mitochondrial dystrophy
Tabes dorsalis (Tabes)
Horner's (H) bilateral
Idiopathic or congenital (I)
MG (M)

Internuclear Ophthalmoplegia

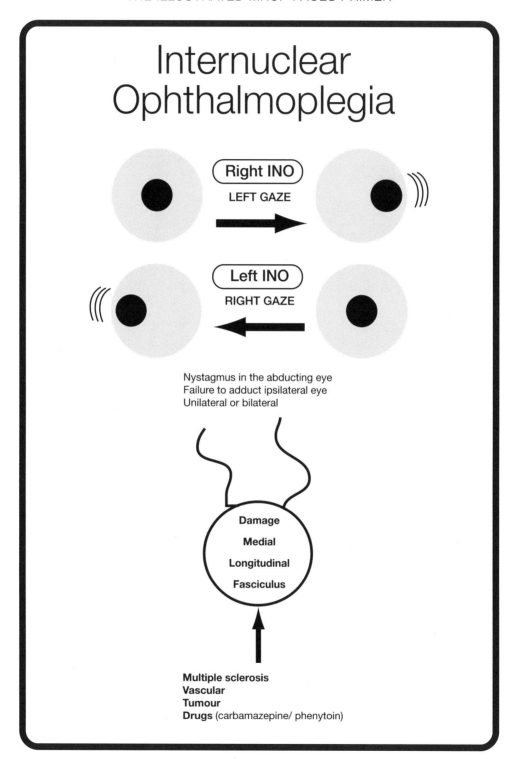

Right INO

LEFT GAZE

Left INO

RIGHT GAZE

Nystagmus in the abducting eye
Failure to adduct ipsilateral eye
Unilateral or bilateral

Damage

Medial

Longitudinal

Fasciculus

Multiple sclerosis
Vascular
Tumour
Drugs (carbamazepine/ phenytoin)

Motor Neurone Disease

Always suspect if combined upper motor and lower motor neurone signs
Eyes, sensation and cerebellum never affected

Pathology of ...

Cranial nerve nuclei

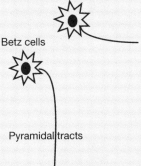

Betz cells

Pyramidal tracts

Anterior horn cells

Both upper and lower motor
neurones affected

Types of classification

Bulbar palsy

Pseudobulbar palsy

 25%

Progressive muscular atrophy

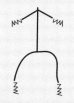

Anterior horn cell lesion
affecting distal muscles

Amyotrophic lateral sclerosis (50%)

Familial version linked to gene
on long arm chromosome 21
– flaccid arms/ spastic legs

Treatment

Treatment
Riluzole (glutamate antagonism) – bulbar
palsy

Monitoring
L-type voltage-gated antibodies for ALS

MRCP specials

Werdnig–Hoffman's disease – causes
floppy infant
X-linked spinal muscular atrophy
Spinal muscular atrophy (chromosome 5)

Multiple Sclerosis

Diagnostic criteria

Clinical: two episodes of neurological deficit at more
    than one site in central nervous system
MRI: T2 shows periventricular white matter changes
VEPs: delayed
CSF: oligoclonal bands

Classification

/\/\ Relapsing remitting

/_/\ Secondary progressive

\ Primary progressive

Features

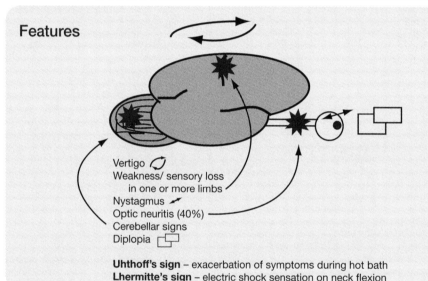

Vertigo ↻
Weakness/ sensory loss
    in one or more limbs
Nystagmus ↗
Optic neuritis (40%)
Cerebellar signs
Diplopia ⬓

Uhthoff's sign – exacerbation of symptoms during hot bath
Lhermitte's sign – electric shock sensation on neck flexion

Treatment

IFN-beta-1a
IFN-beta-1b
Copolymer 1   both reduce the relapse rate in
IV immunoglobulin   relapsing-remitting by 1/3
Steroids for acute relapse
Plasma exchange if no response to steroids
Amantadine for fatigue
Bladder dysfunction: <100 mL – oxybutynin,
    >100 mL – self-catheterisation
Sexual dysfunction: viagra
Limb spasticity: MDT approach

Other demyelinating diseases

Devic's syndrome
Leukodystrophies
Tuberous sclerosis
Schilder's disease

Myasthenia Gravis

Grades (Osserman's)

I   Ocular myasthenia
IIA   Mild generalised myasthenia
IIB   Severe skeletal and bulbar involvement
III   Rapid progression of severe symptoms
IV   Late severe myasthenia – as III but takes two
       years to progress

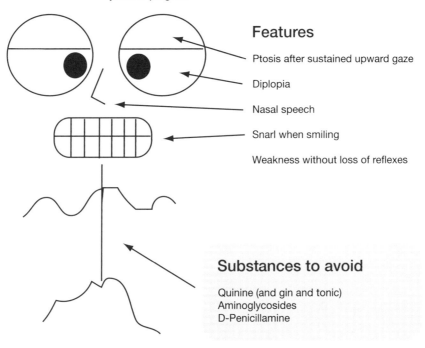

Features

Ptosis after sustained upward gaze

Diplopia

Nasal speech

Snarl when smiling

Weakness without loss of reflexes

Substances to avoid

Quinine (and gin and tonic)
Aminoglycosides
D-Penicillamine

Investigations

Tensilon
Vital capacity
MRI chest
ACh receptor antibodies
EMG (decremental response to
    stimulation)

Treatment

Pyridostigmine
Immunosuppression (steroids/ azathioprine/
    plasmapheresis)
Thymectomy (85% remission with
    improvement taking up to 10 years)

Neurofibromatosis

NFT Type 1 – Von Recklinghausen's disease

On chromosome 17 (Von Recklinghausen has 17 letters)

Criteria for diagnosis

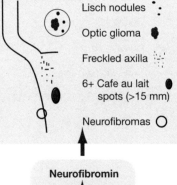

- Lisch nodules
- Optic glioma
- Freckled axilla
- 6+ Cafe au lait spots (>15 mm)
- Neurofibromas

Neurofibromin

17q11.2

AD

NFT Type 2

Criteria for diagnosis

Bilateral 8th nerve palsy on CT/ MR
Unilateral 8th nerve palsy + relative with type 2, + 2 of neurofibroma/ meningioma/ glioma/ schwannoma/ juvenile posterior subcapsular lenticular opacity

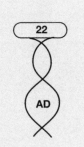

22

AD

G E N E T I C S

Neurofibromatosis associations

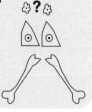

Epilepsy
Decreased IQ
Retinal hamartomas
Lung cysts
Skeletal lesions

Nystagmus

Pendular nystagmus

Eye swings at equal speed horizontally
Occurs with visual acuity defects

Jerky nystagmus = vestibular nystagmus

Central causes

D emyelination
V ascular
D iabetes
T rauma
I nfection
C ancer
S yphilis

Peripheral causes

Acoustic neuroma
Ménière's
Labyrinthitis
Otitis media
Head injury

Dissociated nystagmus

= ataxic nystagmus – irregular nystagmus in the abducting eye

Bilateral

MS
Brainstem tumour
Wernicke's

Unilateral

Brainstem vascular problems

Downbeat nystagmus

Brainstem
Hypomagnesaemia
Meningoencephalitis

Upbeat nystagmus

Anterior vermis of cerebellum lesions

Parkinson's Disease

Causes

Idiopathic
Drugs
Vascular
Post-encephalitic
Parkinson's-plus

Treatment

**L-dopa with decarboxylase inhibitor
(e.g. carbidopa)**
Anticholinergics

Other medications
Selegiline (MAO-B inhibition) – slows
    progression to Parkinson's
Ropinirole (Dopamine agonist –
    decreased dyskinesia risk)
COMT inhibition – e.g. entacapone
    Increases 'on' time
Foetal tissue transplantation
Thalamotomy

Parkinson's-plus syndromes

Steele–Richardson–Olszewski (akinesia, axial
    rigidity, bradyphrenia, supranuclear palsy)

Multiple system atrophy (Parkinson's with
    cerebellar signs and autonomic problems,
    e.g. postural hypotension, bladder
    symptoms, pupillary asymmetry)
    – Olivopontocerebellar syndrome
    – Striatonigral degeneration
    – Shy–Drager
Basal ganglia calcification

Mental problems

Dementia (1/5)
Depression (1/3)
Bradyphrenia
Acute confusion secondary to
    drugs

Upper body dyskinesia

Can't initiate movement
Slow movement
Poverty of movement
Decreased amplitude of repeated movement
Can't do simultaneous tasks

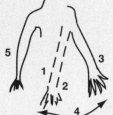

Tremor

3–5 Hz
Intermittent (close eyes and count
    backwards)
Intensified with stress and reduced with
    sleep

Rigidity

Lead pipe rigidity
Cog-wheeling (due to underlying tremor)

NB: Spasticity-clasp-knife/ Gegenhalten or
    paratonia where increased muscle tone
    varies and is worse when tries to relax

The Parkinson's examination

Observe facies → Assess cog-wheeling → Assess thumb to finger speed (bradykinesia) →
Assess gait → Assess handwriting (micrographia) → Look for signs of Parkinson's-plus syndromes

Peripheral Neuropathies

Thickened nerves

C harcot–Marie–Tooth
L eprosy
A myloidosis
R efsum's disease
D éjerine–Sottas'
    disease

Motor neuropathy

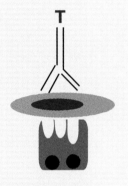

Toxicity (T) (Pb/ dapsone/
    organophosphates)
Guillain–Barré
Porphyria
Diphtheria/ polio
+ Peroneal muscular atrophy

Sensory neuropathy

A myloidosis
B 12 deficiency
C arcinomatosis
D iabetes
E thanol

U raemia
L eprosy

Mononeuritis multiplex

W egener's
A myloidosis
R heumatoid arthritis
D iabetes mellitus
S LE

P olyarteritis nodosa
L eprosy
C arcinomatosis

Dorsal column diseases

Friedreich's ataxia
SACD
Tabes dorsalis

Cerebellar and long tract signs

MS
Friedreich's ataxia
Spinocerebellar disease

Proximal Myopathy

Features

Difficulty standing from sitting
Waddling gait
Look for causes (below)

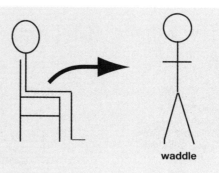

waddle

Causes

G enetic – hereditary muscular dystrophy, i.e. Becker's, Duchenne's, etc.
I nflammatory – polymyositis
E ndocrine – diabetic amyotrophy/ Cushing's/ thyrotoxicosis
M etabolic – osteomalacia
D rugs – alcohol/ steroids/ chloroquine

MRCP specials

Diabetic amyotrophy
Asymmetrical
Absent knee jerk
Sensory loss thigh
Wasted and painful thigh

Pseudobulbar Palsy

Causes

Bilateral stroke
MS
MND

Presentation

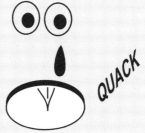

Emotionally labile
Spastic tongue
Sluggish palatal movements

Bulbar Palsy

Causes

Guillain–Barré
Syringomyelia
Poliomyelitis
Nasopharyngeal tumour
Neurosyphilis
Neurosarcoid

Presentation

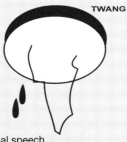

Nasal speech
Wasting of tongue and
    fasciculation
Soft palate weakness
Saliva accumulation

Radial Nerve Palsy

Root values C5 – C8

Causes

Saturday night palsy
Crutches/ trauma
Lead poisoning

Can straighten at IP but not at
MCP if wrist straightened

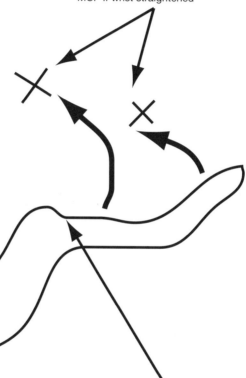

Sensation over first dorsal
interossei decreased

Retro-Orbital Tumour

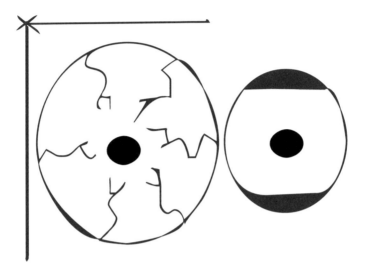

Features

Unilateral exophthalmos
Impaired extraocular
    movements
Chemosis

Causes of unilateral exophthalmos

Retro-orbital tumour
AV fistula
Cavernous sinus thrombosis
Orbital cellulitis

Speech

The speech examination

Comprehension

Put your tongue out
Shut your eyes
Touch your nose
3 stage command

Naming

Pen
Watch

Articulation

'kuh', 'la', 'me', 'ah'
'British Constitution'
'West Register Street'
'Baby hippopotamus'
'Biblical criticism'
'Artillery'

AMTS

Speech problems

1. Dysphasia

Expressive (Broca's area – posterior
   left frontal gyrus)
Receptive (Wernicke's area)

2. Dysarthria

Causes
Local causes (ill fitting teeth, etc.)
Stutter
Cerebellar disease
Parkinson's
PSP
Progressive bulbar palsy

> Cerebellar dysarthria –
> scanning (MS) or
> stacatto (Friedreich's) speech
>
> Test by asking the patient
> to say 'kuh', 'la', 'me' and 'ah'

3. Dysphonia (disorder of volume)

Subacute Combined Degeneration of the Cord

Features

Absent ankle reflexes
Brisk knee jerks and upgoing plantars
Vibration, light touch diminished

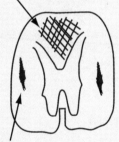

Pathology

B12 deficiency due to:
Decreased intake
Malabsorption: stomach (PA/gastrectomy)
              small bowel (ileal disease/ bacterial
                overgrowth/ coeliac disease)
              pancreatitis
Tapeworm

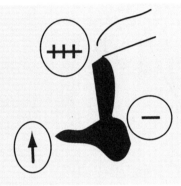

Ascending tracts of posterior column

Descending tract of pyramids

Tests

FBC/ reticulocyte count/ haematinics
IF and parietal cell antibodies
Schilling test
Bone marrow examination

Treatment

For anaemia: Replace B12 before blood as can kill/ make worse
Neurological response to B12 is variable

Syringomyelia

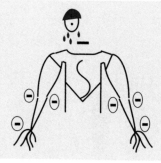

Pain and temperature – cape-like
    distribution loss
Upper limb reflexes absent/ lower limb
    reflexes exaggerated
Hand small muscle wasting + ulnar border
    (la main succulente)
Horner's
Kyphoscoliosis

Pathology

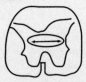

Progressively expanding fluid-filled cavity
    within the spinal cord

Investigation

MRI

Treatment

Syringoperitoneal shunt
Drainage into subarachnoid space
If Arnold-Chiari malformation remove
    lower occipital bone and do cervical
    laminectomy

Associations

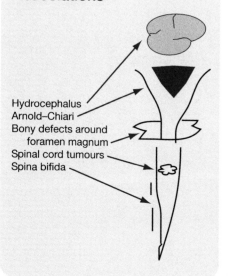

Hydrocephalus
Arnold–Chiari
Bony defects around
    foramen magnum
Spinal cord tumours
Spina bifida

Syringobulbia

Features

Vertigo
Onion skin sensory loss face
Wasted small muscles of tongue
Involvement 5th/ 7th/ 9th/ 10th nerves

Tabes Dorsalis

Features

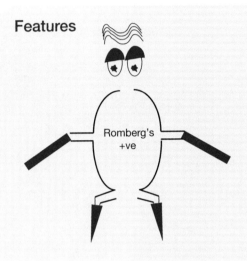

Romberg's
+ve

Frontalis over-reaction

Bilateral ptosis
Optic atrophy
Argyll Robertson pupils

Romberg's positive

Posterior column signs (loss of
        vibration and joint position sense)

High stepping gait

Patterns of neurosyphilis

Meningovascular disease
Tabes dorsalis
Generalised paralysis of the insane
Taboparesis
Localised gummata

Investigation

Syphilis serology (75% positive in tabes)
(VDRL and TPHA)

Treatment

Penicillin V
Lightning pains: carbamazepine
Sensory ataxia: physio
Bladder probs: no anticholinergics/ self
        catheterisation
Ulcers: good shoes
Visceral crises: opiates

Torsion Dystonia

Causes

Hereditary (AR/ AD(9q)/
    X recessive)
Birth anoxia
Drugs
Wilson's
Huntington's
Parkinsonism

Features

Dystonic head and
    neck movements

Blepharospasm

Facial grimacing
Forced opening and
    closing of the
    mouth

Torticollis

Limbs take on
    abnormal but
    characteristic
    patterns

Treatment

Drugs: diazepam/ tetrabenazine/ antiparkinson's
Stereotactic thalamotomy

Ulnar Nerve Palsy

Root values are C8 and T1

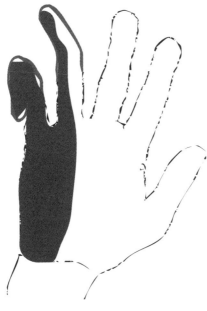

Sensory loss medial one and a half fingers

Supplies ...
Abductor digiti minimi
Flexor digiti minimi
Opponens digiti minimi

Adductor pollicis
Dorsal and palmar interossei
3rd and 4th lumbricals
Palmaris brevis

Test for flexor carpi ulnaris by lying hand palm up against table then asking patient to flex and ulnar deviate at the wrist

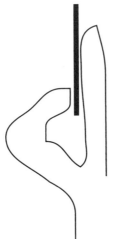

Froment's sign (positive if thumb unable to hold piece of paper without flexing – tests adductor pollicis)

Ulnar paradox – The higher the lesion, the less the disability

Visual Field Problems

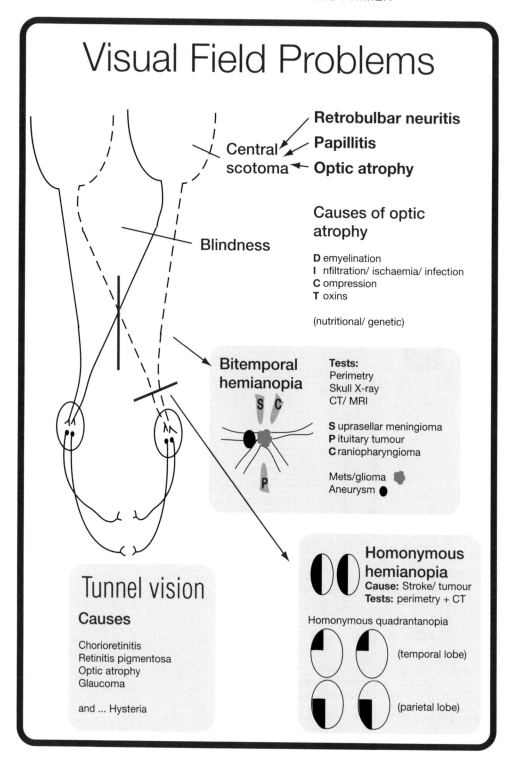

Central scotoma

Retrobulbar neuritis
Papillitis
Optic atrophy

Blindness

Causes of optic atrophy

D emyelination
I nfiltration/ ischaemia/ infection
C ompression
T oxins

(nutritional/ genetic)

Bitemporal hemianopia

S C

P

Tests:
Perimetry
Skull X-ray
CT/ MRI

S uprasellar meningioma
P ituitary tumour
C raniopharyngioma

Mets/glioma
Aneurysm

Tunnel vision

Causes

Chorioretinitis
Retinitis pigmentosa
Optic atrophy
Glaucoma

and ... Hysteria

Homonymous hemianopia
Cause: Stroke/ tumour
Tests: perimetry + CT

Homonymous quadrantanopia

(temporal lobe)

(parietal lobe)

Wallenberg's Syndrome

Pathogenesis

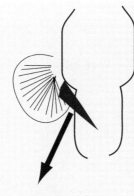

Wedge-shaped infarct
between inferior
cerebellum and medulla

Features

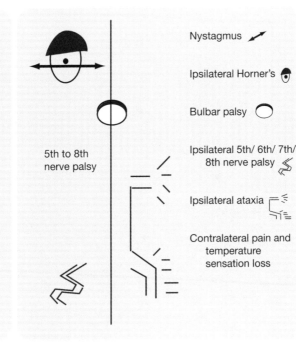

5th to 8th
nerve palsy

Nystagmus

Ipsilateral Horner's

Bulbar palsy

Ipsilateral 5th/ 6th/ 7th/
8th nerve palsy

Ipsilateral ataxia

Contralateral pain and
temperature
sensation loss

Culprit vessels

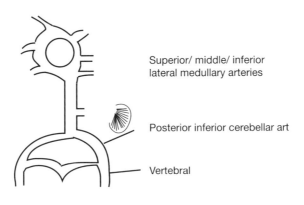

Superior/ middle/ inferior
lateral medullary arteries

Posterior inferior cerebellar art

Vertebral

Wasted Small Hand Muscles

Causes of bilateral wasting

Rheumatoid
Old age

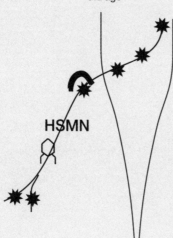

Syringomyelia

Motor neurone
disease
Cervical spondylosis
Bilateral cervical ribs

HSMN

Charcot–Marie–Tooth
Guillain–Barré

Bilateral median and
ulnar nerve lesions

Causes of unilateral wasting

As per bilateral AND

Pancoast's
Brachial plexus trauma
Cervical cord lesion
Malignant infiltration of
brachial plexus

Causes of a claw hand

As per unilateral wasting AND
Volkmann's ischaemic contracture

Respiratory

Asthma
Bronchiectasis
Consolidation
COPD
Cor Pulmonale and Pleural Rub
Cystic Fibrosis
Fibrosing Alveolitis
Lung Cancer
Old TB
Pickwickian Syndrome
Pleural Effusion
Pneumothorax

Asthma

Wheeze differential

COPD
LVF
PAN
Tumour
Eosinophilic lung disease

Management of chronic asthma

Step 1. Occasional short acting
Step 2. Short acting and steroid
Step 3. Short acting + increase steroid or short
　　　　acting + add long acting beta2
Step 4. Add other alternatives
Step 5. Add oral steroid

**Extrinsic asthma
(kids)**
(Dermatophagoides
　pteronyssinus)

**Intrinsic asthma
(late onset)**
Smoking related –
　more severe and
　continuous

Chronic asthma

Wheeze
Cough
SOB

Diagnosis

PEFR >25% variable
PEFR + FEV1 inc post neb
Dec FEV1
Dec FEV1/ FVC ratio
　(<70%)
Gas trapping

Triggers

Infection
Emotion
Exercise
Drugs

Acute asthma

Severe
H R >110
A BG pO$_2$ <8
R R >25
P EFR <50%

Life threatening
PEFR <33%
Exhaustion
Bradycardia/ hypotension

Bronchiectasis

(= chronic necrotising infection)

Types (Reid's classification)

1. Cylindrical
2. Varicose
3. Cystic/ saccular

Tests:
CXR/ HRCT/ sputum culture
Aetiology testing

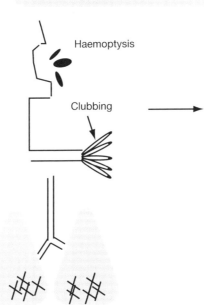

Haemoptysis

Clubbing

Complications

Sinusitis
Haemoptysis
Brain abscess
Amyloidosis
Effusion
Pneumothorax
Pneumonia

Bilateral coarse and end insp crackles – coarse
bronchiectasis. They **c**lear with **c**oughing

Causes

Congenital	Post-infective	Other
CF	TB/ HIV	Sarcoid
Kartagener's	Measles	Aspiration
Young's	Pertussis	Hypogammaglob
	Pneumonia	Idiopathic
	ABPA	

Management

P hysio
A ntibiotics
B ronchodilator
S urgery – if restricted to a single lobe

139

Consolidation

Causes of pneumonia

Community	Hospital
Typical	Atypical
S. pneumo	*Chlamydia pneumo*
H. influenzae	*Mycoplasma pneumo*
	Legionella pneumo
	Chlamydia psittacii

Poor prognosis signs

Confusion and comorbidities
Urea >7
RR >30
BP Sys <90/ Dias <60
Age >65

Extrapulmonary manifestations of mycoplasma

 CNS/ PNS problems

DIC DIC

 Pericarditis/ myocarditis

 Hepatitis
Haemolytic anaemia

 Glomerulonephritis

Dec movement of affected side
Bronchial BS (bronchial)
Crackles ( )
Dec PN – not stony dull (THUD)

Causes of recurrent pneumonia

Aspiration
Antibiotics
Cancer
Churg–Strauss

Pulmonary eosinophilic disorders

Löffler's
ABPA
Chronic pulmonary eosinophilia

COPD

(3 months cough/ year for 2+ years
– a combination of chronic bronchitis and emphysema)

Genetics in COPD

1. Alpha1 antitrypsin deficiency
2. TNF-alpha
3. Microsomal epoxide hydroxylase

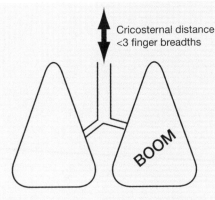

Cricosternal distance
<3 finger breadths

Hyperresonant (and loss of cardiac dullness)
Decreased cricothyroid distance
Decreased air entry

Classification

Mild   FEV1   60–80%
Mod   FEV1   40–60%
Sev   FEV1   <40%

Treatment

Nebulisers/ inhalers/ O_2/ antibiotics

Other treatments

Nutrition (diet high in n-3 fatty acids)
Bullectomy: COPD with >1/3 of hemithorax
    taken up
Lung transplantation: <60 yrs with no
    underlying systemic probs or cancer
Lung volume reduction surgery

Long term O_2 therapy

pO_2 on air <7.3
pO_2 7.3–8 with portal hypertension/ peripheral
    oedema/ nocturnal hypoxaemia
FEV1 <1.5 L
Normal or increased pCO_2

Cor Pulmonale

Mortality 50% at 5 years

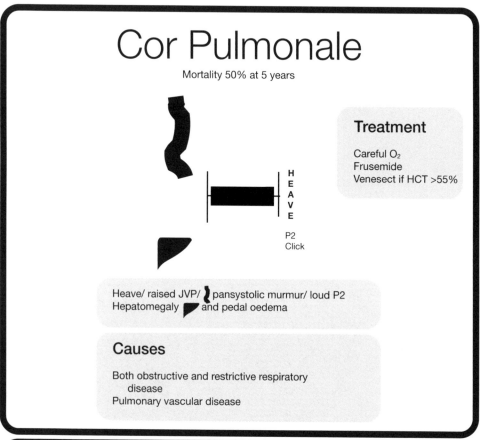

H
E
A
V
E

P2
Click

Treatment

Careful O_2
Frusemide
Venesect if HCT >55%

Heave/ raised JVP/ pansystolic murmur/ loud P2
Hepatomegaly and pedal oedema

Causes

Both obstructive and restrictive respiratory
    disease
Pulmonary vascular disease

Pleural Rub

Causes

PE
Infection

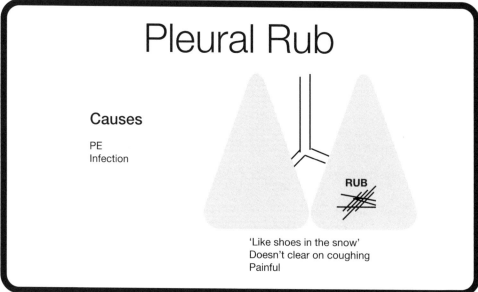

RUB

'Like shoes in the snow'
Doesn't clear on coughing
Painful

Cystic Fibrosis

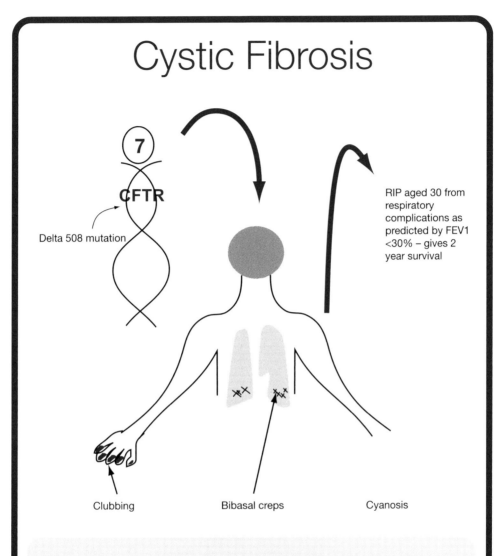

7

CFTR

Delta 508 mutation

RIP aged 30 from respiratory complications as predicted by FEV1 <30% – gives 2 year survival

Clubbing   Bibasal creps   Cyanosis

Treatment

Physio
Antibiotics
Bronchodilators
Heart-lung transplantation
High dose ibuprofen
Aerosolised human recombinant DNase
Improve hydration of secretions with
     amiloride, triphosphate nucleotide
Immunisation

Treatment of steatorrhoea

Low fat diet
Pancreatic supplement
H2 receptor antagonist

Chest infection bacteria

S. aureus
H. influenzae
Burkholderia cepaciae
Pseudomonas aeruginosa

143

Fibrosing Alveolitis

Types

UIP   usual
DIP   desquamative
NSIP non-specific
LIP   lymphoid
GIP   giant-cell

Causes

RA/ SLE/ UC/ CAH/ SS/ dermatomyositis
EAA
Chronic pulmonary oedema
Occupational lung disease

Investigations

CXR/ ABG/ PFT/ HRCT
Inc ESR/ Inc Ig/ Inc ANA/
    RF
BAL: Lymphocytic = good
    prognosis

Treatment

6/52 steroids
Cyclophosphamide for
    steroid non-responders
Lung transplantation – has
    a 60% 1 year survival

Features

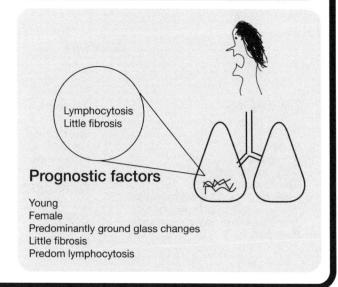

Finger clubbing
Cyanosis
Bilateral fine late
    inspiratory creps
    ('velcro')

Clubbing and creps differential

Bronchogenic Ca
Bronchiectasis
Asbestosis
Fibrosing alveolitis

Lymphocytosis
Little fibrosis

Prognostic factors

Young
Female
Predominantly ground glass changes
Little fibrosis
Predom lymphocytosis

Lung Cancer

Extrapulmonary

Gynaecomastia
TSH raised
PTH raised

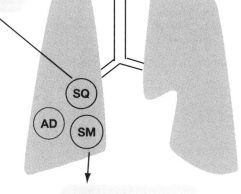

Lung cancer types

Squamous (SQ) and small cell
    (SM) – central
Adenocarcinoma (AD) – peripheral

Treatment

Small cell – chemotx
Non-small cell – surgery/radiotx

Extrapulmonary

SiADH
Carcinoid
ACTH
Eaton–Lambert

General extrapulmonary manifestations of lung cancers

CVS	**Endocrine**	**Skeletal**	**Cutaneous**	**Neuro**	**Vasc**
AF	As above	Clubbing	Herpes zoster	Eaton–Lambert	DIC
Pericarditis		HPOA	Dermatomyositis	Neuropathies	
Marantic				Horner's	
endocarditis				Cerebellar	
				degeneration	

Inoperable disease

FEV1 <1.5 L
Current IHD
Malignant pleural effusion
Mediastinal LN
Carinal involvement

Old TB

Features

Trachea pulled over
May have obvious scar
Creps upper zone

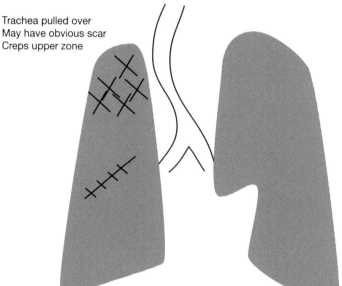

Pulmonary TB diagnosis

If sputum positive AFB: isolation for 2 weeks – can self
   isolate at home
Investigate contacts by enquiry re BCG/ do CXR/ Heaf test
Give chemoprophylaxis if Heaf positive but CXR negative
Early TB diagnosis done by PCR

Pickwickian Syndrome

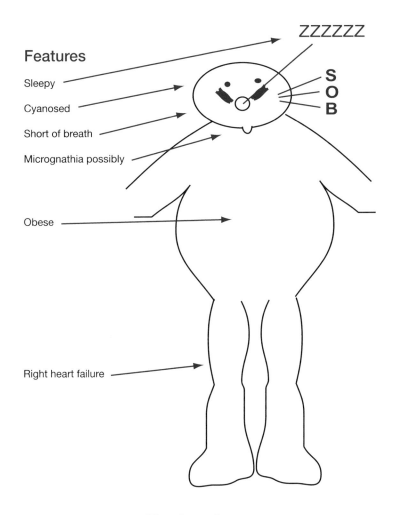

ZZZZZZ

Features

Sleepy

Cyanosed

Short of breath

Micrognathia possibly

S
O
B

Obese

Right heart failure

Treatment

CPAP
Tonsillectomy
Correction of GH/ TSH/ Other
Weight loss
Mandibular surgery
Tracheostomy

Pleural Effusion

Pleural effusion types

Exudate

(Serum albumin: pleural gradient
    >1.2 g/dL = exudate)
Lung Ca/ mesothelioma
Secondaries (breast/ lung/ ovary/ panc)
Pneumonia/ TB
RA/ SLE

Transudate

CCF
Liver failure
Hypothyroid
Nephrotic

Empyema

Chylous

Haemothorax

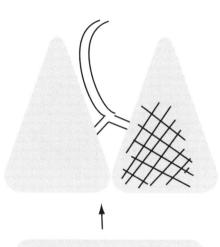

Decreased movement
Tracheal deviation to opposite side
Stony dull
Decreased vocal resonance and
    breath sounds (sounds travel
    badly through water)

Investigations

C ytology: white cells >50 000 – parapneumonia; Lymph – Ca/ TB/ sarcoid/ collagen
P rotein/ pH: If pH <7.2 suggests empyema
G **L** ucose: ↓glu/ ↑LDH – TB/ Ca/ RA/ SLE; ↓glu or ↓LDH – in Ca poor prognosis
Chol **E** sterol: <60 g/dL in transudates
   U
R F: RF and ANA increased in SLE
A lbumin/ ANA/ amylase: Boerhaave's/ bact pneumonia / adenoCa/ pan
L DH

Use of USS

To differentiate thickening from effusion
For drain placement
For loculation

Causes of dullness at the lung base

Pleural effusion
Pleural thickening
Raised right hemidiaphragm
Consolidation and collapse

Pneumothorax

Causes

Spontaneous
Trauma
Asthma
COPD
Ca lung
CF
TB
Ventilation
Marfan's
Ehlers–Danlos

BTS grading

Small (<2 cm rim on CXR)
Medium
Complete
Tension

Dec movement affected
    side
Inc PN
Deviated trachea
Dec breath sounds
If hypotensive/
    tachycardic = tension

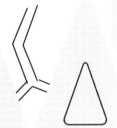
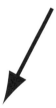

Thoracotomy if ...

a. More than three episodes of spontaneous
    pneumothorax
b. Bilateral pneumothoraces
c. Failure of lung to expand after thoracostomy
    for first episode

Rheumatology

Ankylosing Spondylitis

HLA-B27 associated – siblings have 30% chance of development

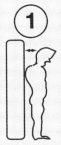 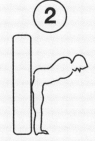

Anterior uveitis
Apical fibrosis
Aortic
  regurgitation
Achilles
  tendonitis

Occiput to wall

Schober's test:
10 cm above dimple of
venus and 5 cm below
If <5 cm separation = failure

Measure chest
expansion

Other seronegative spondyloarthropathies

Reiter's
Psoriatic arthritis
Juvenile chronic arthritis
Intestinal arthropathy

Investigations

X-ray SI joints (erosions and sclerosis)
Radiographs of lumbar spine (Bamboo spine)

Management

Exercise and physio
Indomethacin
Vertebral wedge osteopathy
TNF-alpha blockers

Natural history

40% get severe spinal restriction

Charcot's Joints

Chronic progressive arthropathy due to disturbance of sensory innervation of the affected joint

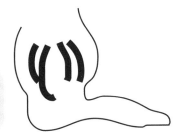

Enlarged
Unstable
Hot and swollen

Causes

Tabes dorsalis
Syringomyelia
Myelomeningocoele
Diabetes
Other (HSMN/ leprosy/
  peripheral nerve injury)

Dermatomyositis

Systemic manifestations

Gut: dysmotility
Lung: cancer
CNS

Investigations

CK+
Aldolase
EMG
ANA
Anti-Jo
Muscle biopsy: necrosis and
    phagocytosis of muscle
    fibres with interstitial and
    perivascular infiltration

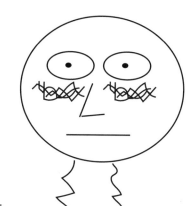

Heliotrope rash

Proximal myopathy

Periungual telangiectasia

Gottron's patches

EMG findings

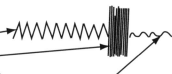

Spontaneous fibrillation
Salvos of repeated potentials
Short duration polyphasic potential, low amplitude

Classification

Group 1: Primary idiopathic polymyositis
Group 2: Primary idiopathic dermatomyositis
Group 3: Dermatomyositis associated with neoplasia
Group 4: Dermatomyositis associated with vasculitis
Group 5: Dermatomyositis associated with collagen vascular disease

Psoriatic Arthropathy

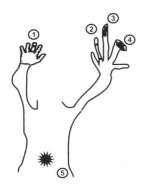

Features

Asymmetric oligoarthritis
Polyarthritis
DIP arthritis
Arthritis mutilans
Sacroiliitis

Investigations

X-ray: pencil in a cup
appearance

Radiology features

Fluffy periostitis
Destruction of small joints
Pencil and cup appearance,
osteolysis and ankylosis
in arthritis mutilans
Non-marginal
syndesmophytes in
spondylitis

Gout

Investigations

On aspirate:
Negatively birefringent crystals
Neutrophilia

Subtypes

Acute
Chronic
Chronic tophaceous

Features

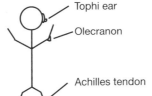

Tophi ear
Olecranon
Achilles tendon

Treatment

Naproxen/ colchicine
(if NSAID intolerant)
Allopurinol if ...
a. Recurrent attacks
b. Tophi
c. Nephropathy
d. Cytolytic treatment
e. HGPRT deficiency

Osteoarthritis

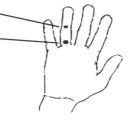

Heberden's node
Bouchard's node

Causes of OA

Primary
Secondary
  Trauma
  Inflammatory
  Neuropathic
  Endocrine (acromegaly/ hyperparathyroidism)
  Metabolic (chondrocalcinosis/
    haemochromatosis)

When talking about management always remember the functional aspects,
i.e. walking aids/ other functional aids and the importance of OT and physio

Rheumatoid Arthritis

Features

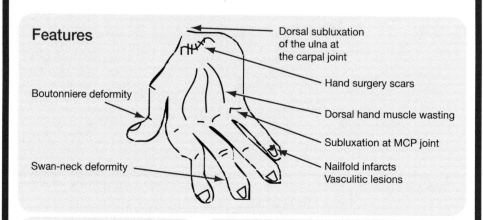

Dorsal subluxation of the ulna at the carpal joint

Boutonniere deformity

Hand surgery scars

Dorsal hand muscle wasting

Subluxation at MCP joint

Swan-neck deformity

Nailfold infarcts
Vasculitic lesions

Prognostic features

Extra-articular
manifestations

Disabled

+RF

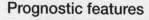

Extra-articular
   manifestations
Disability
Subcutaneous
   nodules
Positive RF   +RF
Insidious onset

Treatment

DMARDs
Aim:
Decrease pain/ swelling/ stiffness
Decrease ESR/ CRP
Correct anaemia of chronic disease
Slow disease progression

Symptom
modifiers

e.g. NSAIDs

e.g. Gold
   Penicillamine
   Methotrexate
   Azathioprine
   Steroids
   Hydroxychloroquine
   TNF-alpha antagonists

NSAIDs (first line. Move to second
   line if no symptomatic
   improvement after 1 month)

Criteria for diagnosis

Morning stiffness for 1 hour for 6 weeks or more
Swelling of 3 joints for 6 weeks or more
Swelling of wrist/ MCP/ PIP for 6 weeks or more
Symmetry of swollen joint area for 6 weeks or more
Subcutaneous nodules
Positive RF
Radiographic features typical of RA

Labs

Increased	Decreased
IgG	FBC
CRP	
CK	
C3/C4	
ESR	

Rheumatoid Arthritis – Extra-Articular Manifestations

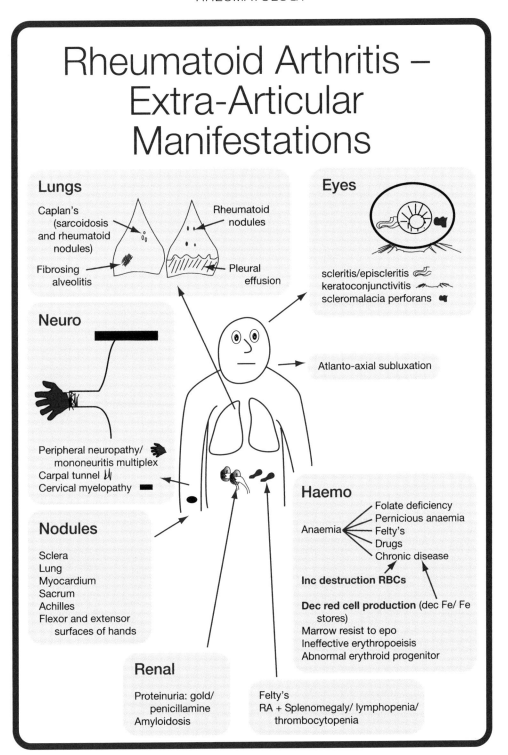

Lungs

Caplan's
  (sarcoidosis
  and rheumatoid
  nodules)

Rheumatoid nodules

Fibrosing alveolitis

Pleural effusion

Eyes

scleritis/episcleritis
keratoconjunctivitis
scleromalacia perforans

Neuro

Peripheral neuropathy/
  mononeuritis multiplex
Carpal tunnel
Cervical myelopathy

Atlanto-axial subluxation

Nodules

Sclera
Lung
Myocardium
Sacrum
Achilles
Flexor and extensor
  surfaces of hands

Haemo

Anaemia
  Folate deficiency
  Pernicious anaemia
  Felty's
  Drugs
  Chronic disease

Inc destruction RBCs

Dec red cell production (dec Fe/ Fe
  stores)
Marrow resist to epo
Ineffective erythropoeisis
Abnormal erythroid progenitor

Renal

Proteinuria: gold/
  penicillamine
Amyloidosis

Felty's
RA + Splenomegaly/ lymphopenia/
  thrombocytopenia

Systemic Lupus Erythematosus

Face
Butterfly rash
Alopecia
Mouth ulcers
Retinal vasculitis

CNS
Psychosis
Chorea
Fits
CNS palsies
Meningitis

Pleurisy
Pneumonia
Pulmonary oedema
Fibrosis

Fingers
Raynaud's
Infarcts in nailfold
Pain (joint)

Renal
Membranous
Crescentic
Diffuse proliferative
Proteinuria

Diagnostic criteria for SLE (need four of eleven)

Malar rash
Discoid rash
Photosensitivity
Oral ulcers
Arthritis – non-erosive
Serositis – pleuritis, pericarditis
Renal involvement
Neurological involvement
Haematological involvement
Antinuclear antibody
Immunological disorder (ANA is positive in 95% of patients. dsDNA positivity is virtually diagnostic)

Investigations

Increased IgG, CK and ESR
Decreased FBC and C3
ANA homogenous
dsDNA (for monitoring)
Anti Ro, La, Sm
Cardiolipin

Treatment

I mmunosuppressives
C orticosteroids
A ntimalarials
N SAIDs
AVOID isoniazid/ methotrexate/ OCP/ HRT/ sunlight
SUPPORT

Systemic Sclerosis

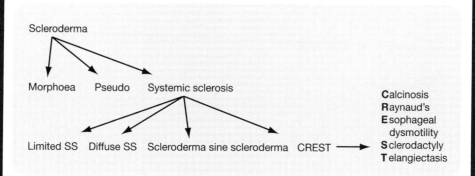

Scleroderma

Morphoea   Pseudo   Systemic sclerosis

Limited SS   Diffuse SS   Scleroderma sine scleroderma   CREST

Calcinosis
Raynaud's
Esophageal
   dysmotility
Sclerodactyly
Telangiectasis

Features

Beaked nose

Telangiectasia

Puckered mouth

Raynaud's

Joint pains

Tight skin over fingers

Subcutaneous calcification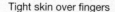

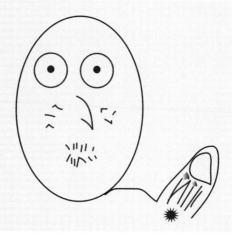

Systemic manifestations

Gut
Dysphagia

Resp
Fibrosis and bronchiectasis

UG
Endarteritis and fibrinoid necrosis

Bloods
Anti-Scl-70
ANA